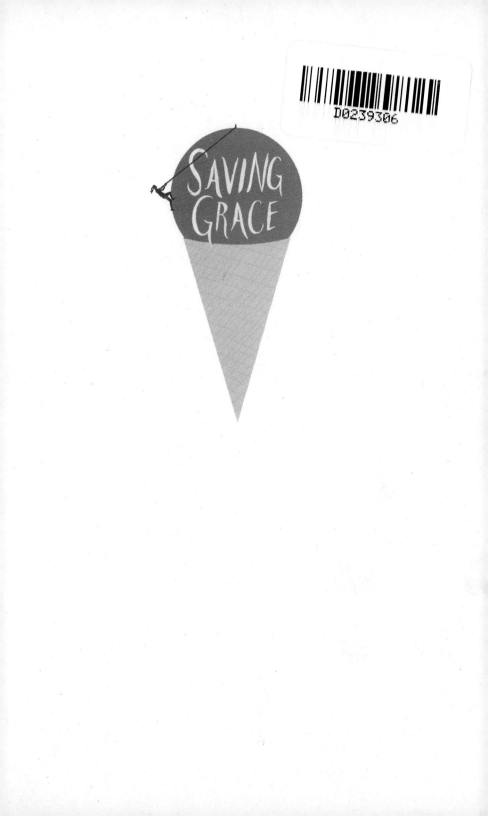

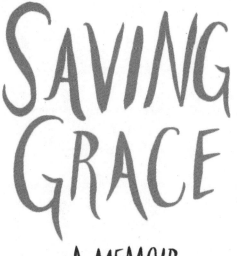

SAVING GRACE

A MEMOIR OF WEIGHT LOSS

GRACE KITTO

september

*To Chris for giving me all the best lines and
Orlando for his support, through thick and thin*

June 2011

Dartmoor is wild and beautiful at this time of year. It's early June and the birds and insects are making a ruckus, a gentle musical hum which fills the air, scented with yellow gorse. Picking my way among the vast rocks, up tangled pathways, through bracken and brambles which catch at my dress, I climb the tor till I'm almost at the top. I'm very fat so it's not easy.

I've heard there's a wild woman who lives in a cave under the tor and rarely comes down or speaks to anyone. I want to meet her. I'm breathless and humbled by the time I get there.

'Hello?' I call into an echoing silence. 'Hello? Bridget? Is Bridget here?' No answer. But in the dark recesses of the cave I see a movement, quick, defensive and silent. She doesn't step forward.

I hang around for a bit but then begin to feel intrusive, as though I'm disturbing her. I turn away and begin reluctantly to make my way down the steep rocky path, stumbling and sliding on the dry, gravel-strewn track.

I become aware that someone is peering after me, and glance back. Two bright eyes dart at me, noticing my every movement. No other word or gesture in my direction. I make my way slowly down the hill, dejected but not defeated. I've glimpsed her. She's seen me and almost acknowledged my presence. I'll come again.

CHAPTER 1

In which the scales fall from my eyes...

17st 6lb

Wednesday, 1 June 2011

I GOT ON the scales this morning full of dread. They shuddered and swung, then settled. I gazed at the result, willing it to be less bad than I suspected. Tears splashed onto my feet because no matter how hard I stared at it, or how I shifted my position, the needle had tipped the next stone and was resting inflexibly at seventeen stone six pounds.

I'm embarrassed that this matters as much as it does. There are plenty of other things in the world to be concerned about – climate change, the arrogance of bankers, the war in Afghanistan, and my son claiming crossly that there's nothing wrong with his school shoes just because they have holes in them and his toes are actually poking through. These things are the stuff of life, they're what I read about and think about and are obviously much more important than this. My weight is just a tiny little side issue, an irrelevance, not important at all in the vast scheme of things. But still it made me cry.

This is not a new problem. In fact, it's wearyingly old. And it's not that I haven't tried to diet. I have, many times. I've lost a bit here, gained a lot there and after years of struggle, have been left with an increasing waistline and a perpetual sense of failure.

It's hard to explain to anyone who hasn't had weight issues where the problem really lies. In my case, there's a disconnect between what I mean to do and what I actually do that stymies me every time. This was forcefully demonstrated by one particular incident a few years ago. I've been mulling on it ever since and trying to make sense of it.

ON THE EDGE of Dartmoor there is a place called Cadover Bridge. It's more than just a bridge. There's a river walk, a picnic spot and a car park all known by this one name. I pass it twice a day on my drive to and from work, a lovely journey across this corner of the moor. Through the seasons I watch the changing landscape of Dartmoor in all weathers, the tors at the horizon on one side and a distant glimpse of Plymouth Sound and the open sea on the other, a twice daily pause for reflection and mental restoration which I love.

It was a sunny day in early summer.

I had a busy production schedule in my job at ITV and during the day had no time to draw breath, let alone worry about my weight. I had finished work and was about to go home. For some reason I can't now remember I started to think unhappily about how fat I felt. I strode across the car park muttering to myself that I was absolutely definitely going to start a diet that very night.

My route home takes me back across the same edge of Dartmoor but with reverse views, obviously. No Plymouth Sound facing this way, but instead I sweep down a long hill towards Cadover Bridge car park, where for eight months of the year an ice cream van is parked. Without stopping to consider I pulled in, bought myself a 99 cone and sat in the car eating it.

Five minutes later I came to, as if from sleepwalking – dammit, I was about to start a diet! I really, really didn't mean to do this. How did I suddenly have an ice cream in my hand? I trembled with frustration and fury at myself. To add to the sense of disbelief, the truth is that I'm not even very keen on ice cream, or indeed chocolate. I don't actively dislike them but neither are my treats of choice.

I couldn't understand how it had happened. Let's be clear, I'm not saying that I blacked out. I can remember buying the ice cream and getting back into my car to eat it. What I have no idea of is how I came to make the decision to buy it, and to override the previous decision to diet. I suddenly saw the complete madness of my situation. No sooner had I decided to lose weight, than I had done this crazy thing. I realised on that miserable sunny afternoon that there were two parts of my brain just not talking to each other. It was as if I was deaf to my very self. It seemed obvious that my unconscious was at work. It had other plans for me that day, not revealed, but demonstrating quite clearly that it was in charge of my actions.

That moment crystallised a recurring problem at the heart of any diet plan I've ever tried. It can't be a coincidence that every time I've made the decision to lose weight, the next thing I know is – bang, I'm suddenly eating a calorie-laden snack that I didn't want and don't need. On that day, at Cadover Bridge, it seemed a clear message that my unconscious was the boss of me. It felt like there was nothing I could do about it.

Years ago, I read Freud as background to a television series I was working on about the history of mental illness. Ever since he popularised the idea of the unconscious, it has been regarded as a powerful force in decision-making. I remembered that according to him, only a very small percentage of our thinking is conscious. On the other hand, the conscious part of the mind is where the verbal self lives, the 'I' we call ourselves. So where had the decision – to eat the ice cream I neither wanted nor needed – come from? My unconscious, I presumed, which was not merely deaf to me, but was cocking a snook at me, having a laugh at my expense. It was maddening.

This is the background to my many failed attempts at losing weight. This was what I knew I had to contend with. I didn't know where to look for answers. I had read a lot about dieting, but nothing that even described this kind of experience. And yet I suspected even then that I wasn't alone and that other people must have this strange, almost out of body experience of eating without having meant to, and then bitterly regretting it. There's something so foolish and self-defeating about it that it's hard to describe truthfully. A humiliating trick of the mind.

Inwardly I named this pattern of behaviour the Cadover Bridge Syndrome. I revisited the incident time and again, trying to understand what had happened to me, not just on that day but on countless days filled with similar episodes. And trying to work out a way of grappling with it.

Why did it matter so much? Because what it demonstrated was a fundamental problem at the heart of my failure to control my eating. I did not experience temptation, uncertainty or doubt about whether to buy the ice cream. I just bought it, ate it and then, only then, came to and regretted it, as if attempting to retract permission in retrospect. This left me in despair. From my point of view, there had been no opportunity for self-control in the whole event. By the time I was aware what I was doing, it was too late. And soon after that realisation the 'sod it' reaction would kick in: if I had already messed up, what's another bag of crisps?! How can you exercise willpower when the rug has already been pulled from under you – by your own unconscious decision-making?

Worse, it made me doubt my own sanity. To decide firmly to do one thing and then immediately do the opposite inevitably leads to self-questioning. The original decision hadn't been half-hearted as far as I was aware. And yet it was repeatedly overridden.

THAT WAS SIX years ago. Since then, nothing has changed except that I've thought about it a lot. That doesn't mean it's been possible to do anything differently. In fact, I've done the same thing, made internal promises and then broken them, over and over again, in a Groundhog Day all my own. And this morning, these shiny digital scales glinting back at me, their electronic numbers trembling and then settling at an ever-increasing weight, is the result.

With a sudden leap of hope, I march to the other bathroom to find my old white Salter scales. I've had them since I was a student forty years ago. They're much more reliable. They have a dial and a needle. I like them. But hope is dashed as they give exactly the same result. Of course they do.

Changing trains at Bristol Temple Meads yesterday, I caught an unexpected sight of myself in a full-length mirror at the corner of an underground walkway. A middle-aged woman, tired, reasonably dressed, but almost square, as wide as I am tall. 'Can that really be right?' I thought. 'Is that really what I look like?' and tried to dismiss it. But couldn't. Hence this morning's weigh-in.

This battle has been going on for most of my life. A memorable statistic for me: aged eleven, I weighed in at eleven stone. I was the height of an adult by then, at five foot four, and a pretty hefty adult weight to match. 'Two Ton Tessie' rang in my ears.

Two Ton Tessie from Tennessee
Holds six sweeties upon her knee
When she does, all the fun begins
When they play tennis on her double-chins

As I got older my (increasing) size sat on my shoulder, ready to bite as soon as things got difficult. Twelve stone aged eighteen, and then down to ten and half as a student, weaving up and down between eleven and thirteen through my twenties and thirties. It's been a long and tricky relationship between me and my body.

There are some things I take comfort in. I've never been a binge eater or a secret eater. I eat with everyone, rarely alone, and not massively more than anyone else, except I've noticed that thin women tend not to have bread when it's handed round in a restaurant, they choose chicken rather than belly pork and refuse pudding. Partly out of irritation with the popular obsession with dieting (or that's what I told myself) I've chosen not to dwell on such trivialities. And now look what's happened.

Looking back with rigorous honesty, I think I've often rooted out the most carb-heavy corner of the menu, kidding myself that I've eaten the same as one of my thinner friends because we've both had a main course, no starter or pudding. But probably I've had twice the calories. She orders lean steak and salad, I have baked potato and cheese. She has fish and steamed veg, I go for quiche and coleslaw.

My husband doesn't know how heavy I am. I can't bear to name a weight of such huge proportions to him. I prefer not to think of it myself, and in fact there is literally no one I will share it with. This is bizarre, because if you ask me what I weighed on any given occasion over the last thirty years I could tell you pretty accurately. That means I've been giving myself an unpleasant running commentary all that time, a critical voice muttering in my head, 'I know what you weigh ...' But there is no one else I can tell.

It's also bizarre, because after all I walk round looking like this every day and people don't spit at me in the street. I'm not a public menace, reviled because of my weight. I have to try to get this thing in proportion, see it in context. There are plenty of other people who have woken up this morning sad to be as fat as they are. Feeling alone with the problem, I try a stretch of the imagination to place myself in someone else's shoes: I could be a student in my twenties who's just tipped ten stone and is devastated, size eight a distant memory. Or a forty-something primary school teacher, her health heading downhill as she hits twenty stone and feels powerless to curb it. Their situations might be widely different but their distress would probably equal mine. The idea of them is comforting in a way – they're fellow travellers – but they don't change my situation.

*

THE QUESTION IS what to do and where to go now? It's a problem, a puzzle, a conundrum. I resist the temptation to set myself an impossible goal: 'I know, I'll get to nine and a half stone by Christmas!' I won't. It's gone way too far for that. This needs to be a radical solution but it must also be achievable. There's nothing more depressing than a goal that's so far out of sight you are defeated before you begin. It must be realistic.

In my line of work, over time, I have had to research a wide range of subjects, and it occurs to me that I can use this experience. I'm not a scientist and I have no medical training so I expect it'll be tough, but it's worth a concerted effort. I will treat my weight problem like a project and try to take the emotion out of it. And I won't talk about it, I'll just do it.

Next, I abandon a timetable for weight loss. It's so tempting to set a deadline – a dress size in a month, a stone before I go on holiday, ten pounds before my wedding ... These goals are hard to achieve and pointless in the larger scheme of things. Yes, pointless.

I'm looking for a radical fix, not a temporary gear change. At work I've got no problems setting schedules for myself and others for months or even as much as a year ahead, so why is it so difficult to adopt the same approach in my personal life? And then inspiration strikes – that's what I'll do. I'll commit now to a year of concentrated effort and see what that achieves. I've no idea whether that's long enough to get me down to a healthy weight or, if not, how much I could possibly lose in that time. It doesn't matter. I'm not going to worry about that now. This commitment is for one year, to see what I can do.

The first thing I need is a simple diet to follow. I'm not setting great store by this choice. After all, the aim is just to eat less food than the body uses in a day, and so burn body fat. It's not complicated. The value of the regime is to help me do it in the most efficient way possible. But crucially, I'm not expecting a diet to fix my mind as well.

Over forty-five years on this particular battlefield I've tried many diets, from high fibre to food combining, the grapefruit diet to Atkins, Slimming World to 1000 calories a day. Here's a secret that not everyone seems to know: they all work. All of them. If you follow them properly, they are all geared to reducing calorie intake and every single one of them will do the job and help you lose weight. But there's the rub of course – *if* you follow them properly. That's the tricky bit.

They each have their pros and cons, but the one I've had most success with from a practical point of view is Weight Watchers. I have some reservations about it because it's a huge corporate concern, designed to encourage increased consumption of Weight Watchers products. The abundance of branded foods and related diet aids bears that out, but the diet itself is good, solid and sane. The WW online programme will give me the food and weight tracking tools I need without having to go to a class, which I've never enjoyed. Result.

But for once I'm clear that picking a diet is not even the beginning of the journey but just a tool, a mechanism to help me on my way. No, the real problem is my mind, which I know will trick me and stumble me, hobble and twist me into repeating the negative patterns of the past. It's my head I must grapple with. I'm going to challenge it, find out what makes it tick, and then work on changing it. After all, you can always change your mind – can't you?

MY HUSBAND AND son don't know I'm doing this yet and I don't want them to. They love my cooking and I love cooking for them, so that isn't going to stop. If I get anywhere, they'll find out soon enough.

'That looks very virtuous. What is it?'

'Just bolognaise. I've done you two some pasta. That OK with you?'

'Sure. Smells great.'

I've adopted a mantra which I chant quietly to myself on the way to work. 'It's only for a year, only for a year.' It makes me laugh. I've rarely lasted three months on a diet since I was in my twenties. Only for a year? Seems like a lifetime. But still I mutter it to myself, as a comfort and a sign of intent. Only for a year.

Sobering fact #1: *Over 63 per cent of Brits and 70 per cent of Americans are overweight.*

National Statistics, 2016
National Center for Health Statistics, 2016

CHAPTER 2

BMI baby

17st 2lb

Saturday, 4 June 2011

THERE'S ONE SMALL piece of comfort. When you're this big, it's actually quite easy to lose weight. By just cutting back a bit, I've lost four pounds before my new diet's really begun. But soon the real Day One looms. I've chosen a Saturday as my starting point. It's taken preparation: shopping, meal planning, clearing the diary of social events involving food.

Last night I signed up to WW online. As part of the process I went through the latest version of their programme, which is constantly refined and refreshed. Having dipped into it many times over the years, I'm familiar with this pattern and knew that I would have to relearn it yet again. To my surprise and relief I discovered that on this new incarnation I can eat as much fruit as I like. It feels like complete liberation and means I will never have to be hungry.

The last time I did this diet, fruit was heavily restricted. There are many people, including my friend Steph, a GP, who say that the fructose (sugar) in fruit will slow down or even prevent weight loss. But fruit is also rich in fibre and I'm assuming that WW has done the maths and decided the benefits of fibre outweigh the negative effects of the fructose. I decide to trust it, and it turns out I end up eating nearly my own bodyweight in fruit daily.

These days I work in a small independent television company where, among other subjects, we make a lot of cookery programmes. When I arrived six years ago it was an almost entirely male environment with a hearty pub culture. Since then, there's been a gradual increase in the number of women employed and the gender split is now pretty even. The atmosphere is bright and creative, and on a good day it doesn't feel like work.

On Monday I go in, determined not to mention my new diet to anyone. By chance, on this day of all days, Molly brings in a fabulous coffee cake she's made and offers it round.

'No,' I snap, and then immediately apologise. 'Sorry, not for me.'

Molly grins knowingly at Anna, 'Oh, she's being good.'

This is an easy response, kind and utterly female, based on the universally accepted formula: not eating equals 'being good'. I swallow my indignation (on behalf of all women – yes, particularly women), smile, and don't have cake.

I've already planned my day's eating so that I don't have to think about it beyond the effort of sticking to it. Recent studies have described soup as an aid to dieting because it gives a sense of fullness without a big calorie load. Years ago, in my twenties, I remember having a lot of success on a diet by simply switching to minestrone for lunch every day. So this is what I'll do: from now on I'll have half a carton of fresh soup each day. I can't cope with the idea of being totally carb-free, so that means half a roll and a tablespoon of low fat cream cheese or a slice of ham too.

Despite having blown my own cover, within minutes of arrival too, I stick to the decision not to talk about my diet at work. It's the kind of thing that the women in the office would naturally natter about, but I fear talking it away. With creative ideas, it's dangerous to discuss them too much because it can prevent you from actually carrying them out. You talk instead of doing. I don't want that to happen with my diet. It feels private and yet, in a heartbeat, two of my closest colleagues have worked out that I'm taking a bit of control – even if they don't fully know my plans.

At home, after only a couple of meals, my husband Chris and son Orlando have guessed that I'm dieting (again), and as usual they're on side. That's great, but I'm still not quite ready to talk it over with them because they've seen me fail so many times before. I'm hoping that this time is different, but who knows?

As much as possible I want to eat with them, and the same food as them, and carry on cooking for them. The answer is to have a light breakfast and an even lighter lunch, leaving room for a fairly normal family evening meal. Thinking it through, I realise that until now I've been eating the same portions as Chris, who is nearly a foot taller than me. In my heart of hearts I've known that isn't right, but haven't been able to stop it. I don't know how I'm going to stop it now.

Orlando is fourteen and for the first time in his life is looking a little plump. I hope it's puppy fat which will naturally melt away as he grows. But my own puppy fat has never magically melted away in forty-five years of hoping. Please let that not happen to him. The last thing I want to do is to criticise him and make him feel bad about his body shape, but I also don't want him to grow up with the same anxieties about his weight that have dogged me about mine. So perhaps I can make some simple changes to our meals that will benefit all of us without banging on about it.

I DO SOME quick research. Body Mass Index is a rule of thumb for estimating body fat based on weight for height. It's worked out by dividing weight in kilograms by height in metres squared. There are plenty of online BMI calculators available. You enter your weight, height, age and gender, and it gives you an index number for your BMI. According the World Health Organization, healthy weight is currently classified as between a BMI of 18.5 and 24.9. From BMI 25 to 30 is overweight and anything above is obese. BMI 40 and above is morbidly obese. I know I should check what my own BMI is now but I can't quite bring myself to do it yet. I'll work up to it.

What I want to know first is where my eventual goal weight should be. The NHS's BMI calculator advises BMI 25, about a pound more than the WHO's BMI 24.9. Crunching the numbers, it turns out that a healthy range for me is somewhere between 8st 13lb and 11st 2lb. This is a shock for starters. So eleven stone is fine for my height? But I've spent my whole life berating myself for reaching eleven stone at age eleven. I hadn't reached full height then so it means that I was definitely overweight but not as drastically as I've always thought. Two Ton Tessie goes straight in the bin.

So where should I set my goal? I like the sound of a BMI of 25, and 11st 2lb seems much more accessible than nine stone anything. But I feel breathless at the very idea. That's over six stone to lose. I wonder in passing how much of that I can shift in a year, but banish the thought at once. That's exactly what I'm not going to do. It doesn't matter. Getting going is what matters.

It's taken a very long time to get to this point. The Cadover Bridge Syndrome played and replayed in my head for a long time after the unfortunate incident with the ice cream and the car park, and I continued to see it in action. I kept trying to understand it. Naming it was good but it wasn't enough. I was hungry for explanation and looked everywhere, scouring diet books and articles, but never found anything that made sense of this pattern of behaviour.

A few years later I finally made a mental breakthrough. I used to have an unreasonable prejudice against the Radio 4 series *In Our Time*. It sounded to me like an extended Oxbridge tutorial and I felt irritated and excluded by it. I'm quite ashamed of this now because I've learned to love it and these days, no matter how random the subject matter, I lap up Melvyn Bragg's Thursday morning offering with relish. This change of heart came about because of the day there was an episode on the fast-developing field of neuroscience.

One of his guests was Professor David Papineau. He described an experiment done by neurologist Benjamin Libet in the 1970s which, he claimed, showed clearly that decisions are made in the unconscious mind before the conscious mind becomes aware of them. Libet asked subjects to do a simple action, such as pressing a button, while electrodes were attached to their skulls, monitoring electrical impulses from the brain. He measured when neuronal activity in their brains changed, indicating that the decision was actually being made. He also attached electrodes to their forearms which measured when the muscle movement took place.

Comparing these two times, his experiments showed there was a gap of about 300 milliseconds (a lot in the field of neurology) between the initial brain activity and the muscle movement which indicated when the conscious decision was made. Melvyn Bragg asked Professor Papineau to explain the experiment in more detail, but the conversation moved quickly and tantalisingly on.

The more I thought about this, the more significant it became. The experiments were simple, but their implications profound. It meant that somewhere in the subject's own brain, the decision to move was busily being made before he was aware of it.

Until then, my knowledge of the theory of the unconscious came, as I say, from reading Freud and Jung as a young researcher. Time to refresh my knowledge.

Freud theorised that our thinking was divided into conscious (about 10 per cent), preconscious (about 40 per cent) and unconscious (the rest). The pre-conscious was a sort of clearing-house carrying messages from the unconscious to the conscious mind via dreams, jokes and Freudian 'slips', inadvertent verbal clues about our underlying attitudes and intentions.

He described the mind as like an iceberg where the larger, unseen unconscious is submerged, only seen at work by its actions. His ideas were based on clinical observation and creative thinking with no physical data to support them, but they caught the public imagination.

Freud's influence can still be felt. There's a loose, shared understanding in our culture about what the unconscious is which owes a lot to his work. But to me it was a very hazy concept until I heard about Libet's experiments. Suddenly, there was proof for the existence of the unconscious mind at work – and it wasn't just an academic construct of Freud's, but could be seen in a series of physical events that were measurable. Perhaps it's a mark of my own pragmatic outlook that this evidence made such a difference to me.

Suddenly the Cadover Bridge Syndrome made sense. My conscious mind had decided on a course of action, but my unconscious didn't agree and had demonstrated its power very forcefully by leading me to the car park, the ice cream and the chocolate flake. It was a light bulb moment. I realised I had spent years attacking the subject from the wrong point of view.

This was a scary idea, because it showed me why I felt so out of control. It was because it was true – I was quite literally not in control. Decisions were being made by another part of myself, largely hidden to my conscious mind. They were being made earlier, too, before 'I' could get a look in. However much I lectured myself about so-called 'willpower', the message was not getting through. The voice in my head was quite literally talking to itself.

That was about three years ago. Clearly, I'm not a fast learner. I wasn't able to process all this, decide on a new course of action and plunge into it straight away. I had to mull some more. Eat some more. Struggle some more.

Everyone has an upper weight limit that they can accept for themselves. For most of us, that maximum gradually creeps up as we get older. In my thirties, my threshold of toleration was about thirteen stone. It's not slim but not massive either. I was lighter than my husband. At that weight I could wear size sixteen clothes and keep out of oversize shops. But middle age has brought a bit more avoirdupois and I've been between fifteen and sixteen stone for the last ten years. That's why Wednesday's weigh-in came as such as shock. The only other time in my life that I've tipped seventeen stone is when I was nine months pregnant with my son and about to pop.

It was careless really. It had been months since I'd checked and in that time, what with one thing and another, I'd acquired another stone. I didn't immediately clock it because I don't believe it's a good idea to weigh all the time. I tell myself that's because I'm not obsessed, but in fact when you have a weight problem like mine, ignoring it is not a good plan. A bit more vanity and attention to detail in that department wouldn't have gone amiss. I might not have accumulated such masses of excess baggage – and, by the way, am I the only woman in the world to take that phrase personally?

However it's too late to worry about how it happened, because here I am and here it is.

A NEW IDEA occurs to me: I need to open a path of communication between the two parts of my mind which are at odds. But how can that possibly be done? Ideas swirl around my head. How can I get in contact with my unconscious?

I try to imagine what it's like.

It is immediately obvious to me that straight-talking isn't effective because, as noted, over the years, I've given myself lectures more times than I can count – result, nada. No, words alone aren't going to work.

I picture my unconscious as near feral, mute and unreachable, so maybe it'll be like getting through to my dog Gina. I'll talk to it but not expect answers and, as with her, will imagine that only one word in ten is understood. I'll try gestures, not too many words. I'll be respectful. Above all, I'll humbly accept that it's my silent, instinctive, non-verbal unconscious that makes the decisions.

If it is indeed in charge, there's no point trying to control it. Instead I'll try to persuade it onto my side. I will not be so arrogant as to insist, demand or declare my intentions. I will humbly request its permission to lose weight. And if it's kindly disposed to allow me, I'll succeed.

This is an epiphany moment. I'm using that tiny scrap of information heard on the radio about Libet's insights to address my weight challenges. It feels cheeky. Here's a beautiful area of intellectual work, still at the cutting edge of psychology and neurology, and I'm just exploiting it to tackle fatness. How humdrum. But if it works, how marvellous.

There's a logical problem right away. If the unconscious is in charge, then even the efforts I'm making now to approach it must have been have been sanctioned by it. But this way madness lies. I can't get into a big existential debate with myself about this. I need to act. So my strategy is simple. I will cast my unconscious as a silent character, like my dog, and talk to it.

My dog Gina is very intelligent – for a Labrador. She lets us know what she wants in gestures. She hints that she's hungry by looking at her bowl, then at me, then at her bowl. She's always fed first thing while one of us makes tea, but almost inevitably when the second family member appears, she'll try the same routine on them in the hopes of getting fed again. She's very convincing, so sometimes it even works. She also has a few dog-words. There's a lot of snuffling and a purr cum growl for love, a kitten-like yelp when she senses that a walk is in the air and a particular sort of donkey bray, which means she's been shut out of the house and wants to be let back in. She's a dog.

Why did I think this would work? Right away I've hit a wall. Casting the unconscious as an animal puts me in charge and it into a subservient position. That won't work because the whole point is that it appears to rule the roost.

Where it is like an animal is that it doesn't speak but is alive and responsive, and I'm trying to communicate with it across a void. But beyond that, the analogy breaks down. From my dreams I can see that it knows everything I know and appreciates the relationship of each part of my life to the next. In them my husband is still my husband, his mother is still his mother and where we live is still where we live. Even if I suddenly dream that we live in Beijing or Buenos Aires, in the context of the dream I know that's a change and an aberration. So however much I love my dog, to treat my unconscious like Gina is to downgrade it. Instinctively I know that respect must be central to my approach and if I think of it as a cuddly black Lab, that isn't the top note. I have to think again.

So on to Plan B: I decide to cast it as a character. What is it like? I don't even begin to know, but as soon as I ask myself the question, a figure pops into my mind fully formed – she's called Bridget. She is slight, medium height, and she has wispy, tawny hair, blue eyes and an air of vagueness. Part hippy, part seer, she lives in a cave under a tor on Dartmoor. She spends a lot of time tending a crackling brazier where she warms herself, and me, and on which she cooks. She couldn't be less like me. I have brown eyes, a thick mop of dark hair, now greying, and there's nothing remotely ethereal about me. I could wish her to be less witch-like but it seems I have no choice. She's already there, in my mind's eye, ready to go.

My imagination roams, trying on all the other avatars I could have chosen. I could have picked a seven-year-old boy called Tom, playing alone in a dusty attic. He would be distracted, charming, childlike, offering naive wisdom. Or Petra, a young librarian with glasses, a chignon and neat suits, preoccupied with her books, with little time for my problems. She would be dry and spare, but full of insight. Or Marina, an ageing mermaid with wonky lipstick bobbing up, every now and then, from the deep. I feel a passing sadness at having to say goodbye to Marina. She seemed like a right laugh. I could hear her giving it to me straight … 'Listen, lovie, what you got to do is …' but it's no good. She fades as I picture her.

Bridget's the girl for me, although I have to fight back a slight reluctance. She's weird, a bit embarrassing, an odd alter ego for someone like me. But I don't have a choice. As soon as I have the idea of her, there she is.

Despite that speed of thought, approaching her is not straight-forward. She's in charge, of course, so she's obviously approved this whole enterprise, but that doesn't mean that she's going to make it easy. She can't speak because part of the problem is that the unconscious doesn't articulate its choices. That'll make it harder to understand her motives and her message. I'll just have to work it out as I go.

Only for a year. Only for a year. Only for a year. I chant it on the way to work, driving over the open moorland. Every time, it makes me smile.

Sobering fact #2: *26 per cent of British people and 36 per cent of Americans are obese, which means they have a BMI over 30.*

National Statistics, 2016
National Center for Health Statistics, 2015

CHAPTER 3

Sweets for the sweet

16st 13lb

Saturday, 11 June 2011

It's my second visit to Bridget and I'm hopeful that I'll actually get to meet her this time. At the entrance there's a door with a narrow grill in it, as if to the gate of a convent. I knock gently, and the grill instantly rattles open. She must have been waiting behind it. I feel foolish, and don't know quite how to begin.

'Could I make an appointment to see you?'

Her eyes are intelligent and comprehending but she seems to feel no compulsion to answer.

'I've got a problem that I'd like some help with.'

A fleeting gleam of mischief in her eyes tells me she knows and is enjoying my discomfort.

'I want to talk to you about my weight.'

I wish she spoke. I stumble.

'Can you advise me?'

The grill snaps shut and as suddenly as she appeared, she's gone, leaving me alone on the hillside, talking to myself. What just happened?

SO, IT'S OFFICIAL. I've begun. Already by the end of a week of carefully following the programme, I've lost three pounds and taken myself below the seventeen-stone benchmark. This is momentous, but it also feels precarious. I still don't want to talk it away because I fear it's a fragile success. I've so often started diets full of determination, only to falter, get distracted, be too busy, go to a special event that means I slip and then never quite get it together to begin again. I don't want to chalk this one up as yet another of those soon defeated episodes.

There's one particular aspect of losing weight which is really hard: that is of course that we have to eat, several times a day too, so what religious people call 'occasions of sin' present themselves on a regular basis. If you decide to stop smoking, drinking alcohol or taking drugs you can be absolute, and abstain. Not so with food. You must eat. That need presents a tantalising series of opportunities to lapse.

All I can do is plan ahead, food-wise, and keep putting one foot in front of the other, ploughing on. Meanwhile, in a spirit of serious enquiry, I think hard about how I got here. Why did I put on so much weight in the first place?

My earliest food memories are from Kenbury, the house where I was born. It was a progressive school run by my parents on the other side of Dartmoor from where I live now. I pass the turning to the driveway from time to time. The house isn't there any more. It was compulsorily purchased and demolished in the sixties to make way for the A38 road to Plymouth. The sadness is that the footprint of the house was several metres away from the road: it never needed to be knocked down at all. But it was.

Kenbury was a dilapidated Georgian manor house of great beauty, of a kind that would be under a preservation order these days. Leaky, rusty, draughty and chilly, it was horseshoe-shaped, with a generous rounded facade and a square back where the kitchen was. From the back door a path led to the crumbling walled garden. There's a scar on my forehead from when, aged three, I clambered along the top of that wall and it gave way, catapulting me onto an upturned slate edging one of the borders.

There were four oval ballrooms within the curved front of the house, two up and two downstairs. 'So oval you couldn't hang a picture,' my mother used to say.

At regular intervals around the front of the house were round-topped windows opening on to the lawn. That style of window still stops my heart, as does the heavy perfume of wisteria in May. One fat, gnarled stem twisted up the wall beside Kenbury's front doors.

My parents, Esther and Francis (known as Fanny), bought the house in a rush of post-war idealism. They admired the work of A.S. Neill, the founder and headmaster of Britain's most famous progressive school, Summerhill. They decided to start a school of their own in Devon based on similar democratic principles.

Kenbury only had about twenty pupils at a time, including my parents' six children, and we were a complete social mix. At one end of the scale were the poorest and most disadvantaged kids in care (the phrase of the time). They were sent to the school by their local authority as a place of last resort because they kept running away from home, were serial arsonists, disruptive, drunken or just impossible to control. At the other, there were posh boys who came to us in a period of confusion and moved on later to public schools. My mother and father welcomed them all, convinced that a mixture of love and freedom would cure all their problems.

They were not the easiest group of kids to live among. A lot of attention-seeking behaviour. They competed for our parents' care and concern, and were usually better at getting it too. We were taught to tolerate all sorts of odd behaviour from them because without exception they had had difficult childhoods.

In the language of the time, they were described as the perpetrators of bad behaviour rather than people who had been ill-treated. These days many of them would probably be described as victims of abuse but in the 1950s they were termed 'maladjusted' and sent away from home. My parents understood this injustice and were their champions with the result that in adult life, out of affection for them, several of Kenbury's ex-pupils took our surname, rejecting their own.

Food was very important at Kenbury. Most people in that post-war period ate what was known as 'meat and two veg' at almost every meal, the vegetables limited to carrots, swede, cabbage and occasionally peas, with boiled spuds on the side. By comparison, we ate impossibly exotic foods: globe artichokes, *aïoli* (garlic mayonnaise before that phrase existed in England), ripe Camembert, aubergines, courgettes and peppers. No one we knew ate like us. My parents had travelled all over Europe and they both loved to cook. They treated it as part of the therapeutic experience. I have photographs of long tables on the terrace at the back of the house, surrounded by adults and children, lolling, talking, eating and lounging around. At this period of my life, food had only positive associations.

On paper it sounds so much grander than it was. There was never enough money. It didn't earn its keep. It was held together by hope. We survived on a wing and a prayer, as my parents used to say, limping from one local authority cheque to another.

Every summer they scraped together enough dosh to take us on long camping trips across the channel to France and Italy, in a Rolls-Royce Silver Ghost. The Rolls was bought from the local scrap yard, bolted onto a different chassis and cannibalised by my father with a truck back, painted white and fuchsia pink, containing the whole school, all of us bonkers children, no seat belts in sight, bouncing around like frozen peas on a sheet of tin. More Larkins than Downton.

This particular story has moved into family myth: one day we were driving through southern France and, towards the end of the afternoon, reached the foothills of the Alps. 'Oh, darling Mont Blanc!' exclaimed my mother, as it loomed out of the darkness ahead of us.

We made our way slowly up into the mountains. Darkness fell and the Rolls strained under the weight of all those bodies crammed into the back. We spluttered to the top but it was becoming obvious that we wouldn't get towards the next town that night, disastrous because my parents were expecting money to be telegraphed to us there. Meanwhile, we were completely broke.

Fog descended just as we arrived at a roadside café for truck drivers. A hazy beam of light blurred by the thickening mist spread across the road in front of us, a real, not metaphorical, beacon of hope. My mother went in by herself and explained our situation, offering our last few francs in return for permission to camp. Half the café tipped out onto the forecourt, their faces blank with shock, to gaze at the strange sight of these mad English people with their ragged children huddled in an open truck-cum-Rolls. Then they started to laugh, roaring and hugging, stamping their feet against the cold, talking fast. We had no idea what they were saying but they ushered us in to the warm café, settled us down on four tables pushed together, and fed us glorious thick onion and potato soup, refusing payment. 'Nectar of the gods,' said my mother.

These are my happiest early memories of food. The way I cook now and even the job I have, as a producer of food programmes, owes a lot to those early experiences. My parents' attitude to eating and indeed life was experimental, open-minded and big-hearted. We ate very well even when we had no money. I don't think that's where the problem began. But then where did it stem from? That's a question I'll return to later on.

MY SUPPER THIS evening is the polar opposite of those rambling, chaotic Kenbury meals. It's counted, weighed, measured. There are strict limits on the amount of fat and carbohydrates it contains. The enjoyment comes not from the food itself, although I make it as appetising as I can, but from the sense of control it gives me to stick to this regime. I do it in hope rather than certainty that it will work.

Finally I steel myself. For a curious kind of entertainment, I visit the NHS online calculator to work out my current BMI. It's 39.4, 'severely obese'. That's just one step away from 'morbidly obese' at BMI 40, where health risks linked to excess weight become very scary reading indeed. These are just a few of them: heart disease, stroke and cancer, osteoarthritis, breathing problems and raised blood pressure.

And then there's my own particular dread, a disease my mother was diagnosed with in her early sixties – Type 2 diabetes. This is what haunts me, if 'haunting' is the right word for something that potentially lies ahead. This is where my fear lies. I watched her gradually lose her sight, sensation, mobility and finally her appetite. She died from kidney failure, the result of diabetes, aged not quite seventy-three. Too young.

I have a photograph of her in my hallway. She used to say that she had a twenty-one inch waist aged twenty-one (quite a contrast to my own spectre of eleven stone aged eleven). From this dreamy black and white photograph of her looking like a 1930s romantic heroine, it's plausible. She was forty when I was born, the last of her eight children, and by then she weighed over twenty stone. I think at her heaviest she reached twenty-four stone.

She was on and off diets throughout my teens, including an early version of Weight Watchers which she encouraged me to join. One of the highlights in those days was a rather dodgy dessert made out of sugar-free jelly and so-called 'cream', which was dried milk powder mixed to a thin paste with a spoonful of water. It was vile, but we thought of it as a treat, an ingenious way to get a bit of sweetness into an otherwise joyless menu. She claimed to have got down to fifteen stone on this diet. It's true she lost a bit, but I'm sure she exaggerated how much. I doubt that she was ever that light as an adult.

Her diabetes was spotted first by an optician who could see changes to her eyes, specifically to the blood vessels on both her retinas. It's a reliable indicator of late onset diabetes. Apart from that tell-tale sign, at that point, aged sixty-two, she was almost symptom-free.

The optician referred her to her doctor, who confirmed the diagnosis. He arranged for her to do a daily finger prick test to monitor her blood sugar levels. Understandably, her first reaction to the disease was panic and dismay but she very soon got used to the idea, so much so that she ignored warnings about its likely progress and took almost no evasive action – no more diets, no exercise. She would diligently carry out the daily blood test but every morning, without fail, would emerge from the bathroom looking pleased with herself. 'Spot on!' she would call out.

Her cheery manner signalled that she didn't need to make any changes to what she ate that day. She felt free to pack in as much carb and fat as she liked, which was a lot. She seemed to be wilfully blind to the dangers of the condition. I don't want to repeat her mistakes and yet I've been wilfully blind to my own situation for over forty years. That's a very long time to learn bad habits. When I think about it, what's changed that means I can tackle it now?

The answer is that I'm here, writing about it, telling you, telling myself. Actually thinking about it, instead of letting the words slide by. I need to take it in and act upon it. Otherwise I'm like a smoker with emphysema, taking a sneaky drag on one more wicked ciggie. I have so often mouthed the words that appeared to commit me to change and self-control, only to fail in the long run to act on them.

None of this is about self-criticism. It will sound like that, but I'm well aware how I've made my choices. In a nutshell, I have overeaten all my life because I felt literally unable to do anything else. There are far more factors in play here than just the role of the unconscious or indeed my family history. Exterior pressures have a major influence too. Try for starters the role of the food industry and its overuse of sugar, salt and fat. The prevalence of cheap unhealthy fast food. Yes, I know, you don't have to eat it. But have you ever taken a four-hour train journey to London and really looked at the food on offer? There is nothing a healthy eater would want to consume.

Equally this is not about fat-shaming. I'm not in the business of throwing brickbats or blaming anyone for their obesity, myself included. But for me, this weight is too much. It's not comfortable, not pretty and I don't need it any more.

Writing this diary is my attempt to untangle the knot at the heart of the issue. It has so many strands, stresses from inside and pressures from outside, that it's hard to be clear about the factors at work. It's all muddled in my head. But if I want to change, I have to question and unpick. And I do want to change.

I have a new mantra to remind me where I was when I started. I chant it on the way to work: 17 02. 17 02. 17 02.

As you see, I've already blotted out the four pounds I lost before I signed up to WW. It's like it never happened. We won't speak of it again. This is my starting weight now. 17 02. 17 02. 17 02.

Sobering fact #3: *Currently, 90 per cent of adults with Type 2 diabetes are overweight or obese. People with severe obesity are at greater risk of Type 2 diabetes than those with a lower BMI.*

Public Health England, 2014

CHAPTER 4

The plan shapes up

16st 10lb

Saturday, 18 June 2011

Bridget is sitting on a stone, next to an open fire. She's gazing into its depths, willing me to go away. This is the first time I've seen her clearly. She's small and her tawny, flyaway hair partially obscures her face. Her eyes, unlike mine, are blue. It's a good colour for gazing into the middle distance.

I realise that I'm intruding but am determined to persist. This time I decide to try being quiet as a way of communicating with her. I sit down opposite her without speaking and I gaze into the fire too.

This is companionable as far as it goes. But it's limited. There's not much I'm going to learn if I can't speak and am not spoken to.

After a little while I get up to go. I can't decide if it was worth it or not – the long trek up to the tor, the sitting in silence, the tenacious waiting.

'Bye,' I call, hoping for a sign of recognition.

She glances up with a swift, mischievous smile. I am quite suddenly completely charmed.

WHY ARE WE so guarded about what we weigh? In our culture, for most women it's even more taboo than discussing what we earn. My husband asks and I refuse to tell. I promise to let him know when I'm lighter than him. This is ridiculous when you consider that he sees what I look like every day, sleeps next to me every night and is well aware of my physical shape. So why is putting a number to it so threatening? I don't know, but I'm not tampering with my state of mind at this delicate moment so I keep schtum. He'll have to wait.

My friend Angie is obsessed about her size, which is actually quite modest by my standards. She keeps up a near daily running commentary. 'I'm fat as a Sumo/fat as a hog/so fat I can't see my feet.' She asks for constant reassurance that she's not as fat as she feels, but brushes aside any comfort offered. She weighs every morning, and sometimes at night too. Some days she declares, 'I've put on pounds! In one day! It's not fair.' I try to be supportive, but the dramatic swings of mood are hard to keep up with. And anyway I'm busy keeping up a steady momentum of my own.

I've lost another three pounds since I started the WW plan and am quietly pleased with myself. It's tempting to think, 'This is so easy – why didn't I do it years ago?' but I make an internal promise *never* to say that. I didn't do it because I couldn't. If you are trying to do it and you can't, forgive yourself. Listening to your own internal critic on this issue in particular is not constructive. In fact it's possible that it's actually part of the problem. We seem programmed to judge ourselves constantly, and to find ourselves wanting. It's no wonder rebellion kicks in, and the unconscious refuses to comply. So never imagine that this is just a question of willpower, whatever that is. It's much more complicated than that.

It occurs to me that one of the most essential qualities needed to lose a lot of weight is patience. Sometimes we feel hungry, and we must wait to eat. Sometimes we want results, and they're slow to come. Personally I'm in it for the long game.

I think about my job. The degree of detail needed in our schedules at work is amazing – who'll be on a shoot in Oxford in the middle of November, and who'll be on leave at a wedding; who'll be preparing for an edit in September; who's going to fly to Scotland for a meeting with a presenter; where I'll be on 6 June next year. At the beginning of a big production it can feel overwhelming, but experience shows that chipping away at it, bit by bit, gets the job done. Human beings seem programmed to comply – the trickiest-looking schedule is made possible by simply chugging through it. If I can do that for so many people at work, myself included, then surely I can schedule my own weight loss journey to be just as slow, considered and achievable. Step by step, that's the key.

Most diets recommend a weigh-in once a week. In theory that feels about right, although it's hard to resist jumping on the scales every morning. But I know that if I weigh every day I'll see natural fluctuations which mean very little and could make me lose sight of the long game. I decide to concentrate on two perspectives:

1. What can I lose *this week?* That's to keep my eye on the ball in the short term, and
2. What is my overall goal? Which is of course a BMI of 25.

Anything in between those two timescales isn't worth worrying about. I've often heard people trying to force themselves to lose a specific amount by a particular date: half a stone per month, or ten pounds before the summer holidays – yadda, yadda, yadda. That isn't planning, but planning to fail. It suggests a degree of control that we simply don't have. We can only control our eating, not our weight loss. To pretend otherwise is to court disappointment. The principle I'm working on is that if I take care of the ounces, the pounds will take care of themselves.

THE ACTUAL RHYTHM of the diet is working well. Breakfast is the same every day. It includes one piece of bread (all the bread I'll eat most days), protein and fruit. It excludes butter. Although I love it, I've decided that for the duration of my diet it's a luxury that I will normally do without – an occasional treat.

Soup for lunch is perfect. I've adapted so well that I soon abandoned the half a roll and cream cheese that seemed so essential on Day One. At that point, the idea of going without some form of carbohydrate at midday panicked me. 'Panic' sounds ridiculous, disproportionate, but it's true. I actually felt anxious at the thought of not eating carbs at lunch. Now I see that I don't need any and I'd rather save those calories to eat at home in the evening with my family.

Luckily both Chris and Orlando like vegetables because my eating plan is packed with them. I make a big herby salad with hot chicken strips for Chris and me and cheese for Orlando, who is vegetarian, no carbs for anyone. I worry it's a bit spartan but in fact it turns out really well, fresh and full of flavour. They follow theirs up with a slab of chocolate each. I don't.

Temptation looms. There are low calorie hot cross buns in the bread bin (who bought them? Me, of course) and I fret about whether to eat one or not, convinced that a small bun at this time of night would make me feel happier. But it wouldn't. It's not worth it. I can do this. Half an hour of self-distraction sees off the urge. I go to bed, happy to abandon any more meandering thoughts of what I can eat until tomorrow.

This is a therapeutic technique called 'distress tolerance'. It's aimed at mood management. The idea is that however miserable you are, however much you want to eat, drink or whatever other self-soothing behaviour you are tempted by, if you wait about fifteen minutes, the feeling usually subsides. Your emotions change, even when you're totally convinced they won't. When the going gets tough it's useful to remember this.

Remarkably, my colleagues – the women anyway – have already started to notice my weight loss. It's only half a stone and I've kept quiet about it, but one by one they mention it, and are kind. I shrug it off. 'Oh I'm just having a dabble,' I say, 'giving it a go.' It's noticeable that my male colleagues aren't nearly so attuned, or possibly they feel less able to comment.

Perhaps many (most?) women share anxieties about their own body shape which keeps them sharp and observant. As a leftover eighties feminist, I'm ambivalent about this. On the one hand I think we shouldn't have to care as much as we do about our bodies, women are programmed to be anxious about their looks and are judged too much by them, it's everyday sexism. On the other hand, I take a pragmatic view: I need to lose weight to stay healthy.

It seems that the whole subject provokes conflicting emotions in us all. I keep tripping over other people's worries, shared in rushed conversations at the shop, on the dog walk or in the kitchen at work – 'I worry about what I'm eating every day', 'I never weigh myself because I'm scared of getting obsessed, but my clothes feel tighter and I hate it', 'it's wine in the evening that whacks it on for me – but I only have a glass or two, and I don't feel as though I can give it up'.

One of my own trains of thought surprises me: shame. Not the shame that you might expect, i.e. how did I let myself get so out of hand in the first place? No, what I'm talking about is a distinct tinge of shame connected to what I'm doing now, that I'm tackling it, that I still care, that I'm still preoccupied with an issue that's bothered me since I was ten.

Sal and Daisy, two of our young researchers, raised this with me the other day. One of them asked, somewhat wistfully, 'Isn't there a time in life when you can stop worrying about what you eat and what you weigh?' The other sat nodding in agreement, willing me, I thought, to reassure them. The fact that at my age I am still occupied with this very issue seemed to ramp up their anxiety. Clearly they wanted to hear that they would reach a point when it wouldn't matter and they could consider themselves off the hook. My answer is that of course there's a time when enough is enough. There is such a thing as thin enough – and a BMI of 25 is a good place to start. In middle age it's no longer about looks and attracting a mate but long-term health and well-being.

Emotions and gender politics swirl around this topic but I decide not to address them all, or try to deal with the problems of the wider world. I'm just going to keep my head down and keep going.

At the same time I adopt a new exercise for the daily challenge of how to control eating between meals. Breakfast and lunch are easy because they're pre-planned, but there's a danger point in the late afternoon when I'm hungry and not due to eat for an hour or so. Also, it's easy to stay on plan for supper but the evening afterwards is full of temptations.

My new idea is this: self-deprivation doesn't work, so I'm going to give up saying 'no' to myself. That probably sounds risky, but there's a caveat: I'm going to manage the problem by simply increasing the amount of time between deciding to eat something, and eating it.

For example, I'm very fond of a mint biscuit called a Viscount. It's counted as only two WW points per biscuit and I work out that I can fit two a day into my diet. I take them from the packet and place them on the table. Have a cup of tea, play a game of Scrabble with my husband, chat. Eventually I eat one. It's delicious. I take small bites, and savour it. Finally I have the second one. Don't read, look at a computer, listen to music or talk. Don't eat distractedly. Enjoy it. Then that's enough. I'm gradually increasing the time between the decision and the act and it begins to feel as if I can take control. It's like developing a muscle. It gets more comfortable. Eventually I'll put off the moment of eating so long that I'll decide not to bother.

I've spent years avoiding Viscounts like the plague because although I love them, they're calorie laden. Now I embrace them. I eat a packet a week and I'm still losing weight. Magic.

Later I stumble on an online article which suggests there's a name for this approach: mindfulness. It originated in Buddhist teaching and breathing meditation is one of the core components. The idea is to become more aware of the body's natural rhythms and to create a sense of space in the mind. It's increasingly popular in the west as a means to treat stress, depression and anxiety. I wish I'd discovered it years ago. In relation to food, the essence is not to eat on auto-pilot but to be conscious every step of the way, to savour, to do it deliberately, to fully notice when you're hungry and to reconnect with the decision to put food in your mouth.

When I was fourteen I made a cheese sauce one day and something inspired me to stir into it stiffly beaten white of egg and then bake it. I was astonished when it rose, light, airy and exquisite. My mother was full of praise, and to my astonishment boasted to everyone about my achievement.

'Delicious cheese soufflé, darling! I had no idea you knew how to make one. Who taught you?'

She was jubilant, but I was crestfallen to hear that my dish already existed, and had a name. I've never quite recovered from the impression that I did in fact invent it. Mindfulness falls into the same category. There I was, devising what I thought was a brilliant new strategy and it turns out it's already been in existence all along. The consolation is that its growing popularity reassures me that this approach is valid, effective and good.

Settling into this new regime is not as hard as I thought it would be. From a physical point of view, the number of calories (points) I'm encouraged to eat is generous so there's no need to feel hungry or deprived. On the mental side, I'm working hard on a change of perspective. Cautiously optimistic, you might say.

Sobering fact #4: *29 million people in the UK tried to lose weight in 2013.*

Mintel, 2014

CHAPTER 5

In which I plateau at week 3

16st 10lb

Saturday, 25 June 2011

Bridget seems to be playing cat's cradle by herself. She sits in the early summer sun on a huge rock, red and yellow wool loosely wound on a spool, spilling around her. I would say she's knitting, but that would be overstating it. She's fiddling about with coloured wool, and looking purposeful.

'Hello.'

She looks up, expectant. Then back at her wool. I can't work out what she's trying to do with it.

'Are you busy?'

She raises her eyebrows. Dumb question. She's always busy.

'I wanted to ask you about what I'm doing.'

I think I see a twitch, an impatient shrug, as if to say, 'Here we go ...'

'I thought you might know why I've stalled?'

She looks straight at me. I get the uneasy feeling that she'd like to say, 'It isn't all about you,' but of course she doesn't utter.

I'm indignant, as though she's spoken.

'It *is* all about me – it so is! That's what I'm here for. How can you think it isn't?'

At which she picks up her knitting and stalks off. One thing's for sure – there's no arguing with her.

NO WEIGHT LOST. I'm resentful and childishly feel it's unfair. Plateaus we expect – but in week three? That's unreasonable. I've followed the plan to the letter and cannot understand how the scales are staying resolutely fixed at 16st 10lb. But it doesn't shake my resolve, although I don't know why it doesn't. In the past, disappointment has often led to a quick slide. Maybe the difference is that this time I'm not letting myself get away with it. I committed for a year, so what's one week of poor results? Nothing.

I saw a blog this week posted by a student who had lost ten pounds and then hit a plateau. She was very dispirited. I wrote back to ask if she had read her own entry. 'You've lost ten pounds dammit, that's brilliant. When you look back at your total weight loss this time next year you won't care which week you lost which pound in.' I could have been writing to myself.

As I sit here writing, I long to eat. I'm ashamed to admit it. On the virtuous moral high ground where I've positioned myself, pontificating away on my computer, the sensation is at odds with what I'm writing. Here at the keyboard I'm in a perfect world, for the time being, in control of my food intake, no need for greed or hunger. It would be such a pleasure if it was all this straightforward, but of course it's not. A perfect world doesn't allow for feet of clay, or human frailty. The reality is that sometimes I will be tempted to slip and sometimes I will. Reality bites – and I bite back, right into a slice of pizza.

A quick aside on the notion of the 'slip'. This is a phrase used in Alcoholics Anonymous to describe a relapse, usually temporary, after a period of sobriety. For AA members, any alcohol intake at all qualifies as a 'slip'. Normal eating, on the other hand, is just moderate consumption, not total abstinence, so does the idea of a 'slip' make any sense in that context? I think it does. We all know what healthy eating looks like. And it doesn't look like cake.

I realise that this sounds obvious but believe me, inside my head, it isn't. I often struggle to convince myself that this one little cupcake in front of me now really matters, that eating it will actually do harm. And yet it is the many cupcakes denied along the way that do make the difference in the end. And before you exclaim and object, yes of course there will be a day when eating one every now and then won't be a big deal. But not today.

Despite the stalling this week, my tentative steps to connect with my unconscious seem to be reaping rewards – six pounds off so far.

I LISTEN AGAIN – and again – to the same 'Neuroscience' episode of *In Our Time*. Melvyn Bragg sounded as interested as I am in what Libet's experiments showed, but his guest, Professor David Papineau, having raised the topic, admitted the results were 'contentious' and moved quickly on. Presumably he meant that they've been criticised because the methods and technology used were crude by contemporary standards.

Scanning the web, there are lots of references to Libet's work but the current picture is confusing, probably because the field is developing so fast. It takes time for ideas to filter from academia to the world of us mortals.

Hungry for information, I search for more details about Libet's actual experiments. He carried them out in 1966, five years before the first digital clock was invented. That must have made it difficult, to say the least, to measure a 300 millisecond gap between the unconscious mind deciding to act and the conscious mind catching up.

In the absence of a digital device, he set up a cathode ray oscilloscope to record data as a dot travelling in a circular motion, in effect, like a clock face. Each participant was asked to look at the moving dot on the oscilloscope and note its position when he or she decided the press the button.

Libet could therefore estimate the time gap between these events pretty accurately even in a pre-digital age. Ingenious. He showed that neuronal activity was taking place 300 milliseconds before the conscious decision to press the button was made and that another 200 milliseconds elapsed before the actual pressing of the button.

In recognition of his work Libet was presented with the first ever Virtual Nobel Prize for Psychology, an award invented to make up for the fact that there is no genuine Nobel Prize in this field. I am moved on his behalf, and raise a virtual glass to his success.

Benjamin Libet's work sparked off a huge debate among academics about the role of the unconscious and the nature of free will. In a nutshell, the question was – if decisions are made by your unconscious before you even know you're deciding something, then how much power does your conscious mind have? Who is really in charge? Not the voice you hear in your head, even though it's telling you it makes all the choices.

This is so pertinent to me and to the Cadover Bridge Syndrome that I'm giddy with excitement. Looked at in one way, the implication is that there's nowhere to go, that we are all at the mercy of an unreachable part of our own brains. That would be the negative way to look at it. I take the opposite view. What excites me so much is that at least it begins to offer some explanation. It stops me feeling that I'm completely insane for eating that ice cream. If I begin to understand, then surely I can learn to change.

CHRIS IS THE person I would normally discuss research like this with because he reads more about science than I do. In this house we say he's better at the green questions. But we circle around each other, not going there. I know of old that he finds it hard to congratulate me about early success on a diet, probably because I've so often failed in the long run. And right now that's fine by me, because it feels like my project.

When Chris wants to lose weight, he just gives up beer and digestive biscuits (two favourites, but not together) for a few days. If hunger pangs hit him at bedtime and his stomach rumbles, he says 'good' and goes to bed. He welcomes it as a sign that he's on track and seems to have no other emotional baggage about the issue, which is remarkable to me.

I've never been able to react the same way. In the past, when I've been on a diet and got to that same uncomfortable moment of the day, and complained, he would say 'good' and turn over to go to sleep, meaning, I suppose, to encourage me to see it as a positive thing in the same way that he did. I would laugh, but feel a little sting of pain, like an elastic band pinging, a mild sense of outrage that he didn't understand I was really suffering.

This diet is different. For the first time in years, this struggle is my own. I don't want to involve him in it. There's something private about these first weeks which I put down to the fact that I've actually faced that it could take a year. A long time, but paradoxically, as a timescale in which to change your whole life pattern and reap such rewards, it's the blink of an eye.

Being overweight is infantilising. Outsize clothes are tent-like and lack definition, like overgrown baby clothes. More than that, I sometimes feel that being fat is like wearing a badge that says you have a massive lack of self-control.

I mention this to Chris who horrifies me by agreeing, a bit too readily in my view. He says that whenever he meets a fat person he thinks, 'What's your problem?'

This is interesting. I've been a fat person nearly all my life and felt the sense of public humiliation that it involves – it's an outward admission of inner turmoil. But I had no idea he thought that way. It seems hugely unfair to me.

'Are you seriously telling me that you think thin people don't have just as much baggage and just as many emotional issues as fat people?' I ask him. I'm indignant, stuttering with rage at this idea.

'You don't think thin people have areas of inadequacy too? That's not fair. Just because you can't see their problems, doesn't mean they aren't there.'

He agrees – in theory – but sticks to his guns. He says he looks at overweight people and immediately asks himself what's the monkey on their back. It doesn't matter how often he repeats it and how many different ways he finds to say it, I don't like it.

Taken to the extreme this suggests to me that he thinks he (thin) is somehow more capable, resolved and functional than me (fat). I bite back the temptation to retaliate and share some of his deficits with him. But this is not a competition. I try hard to understand what he means, and unfortunately I can.

How very annoying.

Sobering fact #5: *Most diets claim weight loss of 1–2 pounds per week is achievable, but research shows this is an unrealistic expectation.*

National Institutes of Health, 25 August 2011

CHAPTER 6

To look like everyone else

16st 8lb

Saturday, 2 July 2011

'Look, what I've come to say is … well, it's a bit awkward.'

Bridget tends the fire, poking about among the ashes with a stick.

'I think you might believe that you're protecting me. Is that it?'

She looks down, drawing the embers together into a neat pile. They catch again, smoking and sparking into life.

'I feel as though you think that being fat is good for me in some way, keeps me safe, comfortable, wrapped up. Is that right?'

She gazes intently into the flames. I try to catch her eye but she won't look up.

'I want to say that it isn't. Good for me, I mean. I don't need it any more.'

An almost imperceptible shrug, as if to say that she would be the judge of that.

'I don't want it. It causes me pain, and it's bad for me. That's all.'

Without waiting for acknowledgement, I turn and trudge back down to the village. I'm glad I've made my point but I'm under no illusion – if she doesn't agree, it won't make a bit of difference.

———

THERE'S SUCH A lot of stupid stuff written about obesity. Column inches about spare inches. It's hard to stomach, and yet we gobble up magazine articles and photo spreads which purport to let us into the 'secrets' of weight loss. Me too, I must admit, but they make me mad.

There's the great 'before and after' photo scam, in which celebs who don't really have a weight problem but do have exercise videos to sell, or a diet to promote, suddenly allow blubbery photos of themselves to appear next to 'transformation' pictures showing them svelte and gorgeous. They are irresistible, but pernicious. They keep us hooked on the idea of a quick fix to dieting, which is palpably nonsense. I know that, and yet I read them.

This week I bought a mainstream (not diet) glossy magazine purely because it was themed around weight loss. I could not believe the quantity of tosh it contained. Two photos of a famous footballer's sister dominated the front cover. In one, she looked pretty large in a scarlet dress which barely contained her. In the other she was a bit smaller, squeezed tight into leopard skin, captioned as 'a slim 11st down from 14st'.

I looked closely at it and found it hard to believe that either of those weights was accurate. At a guess, I'd bung two stone on to both the 'before' and 'after' photos. Why lie? I imagine because that was part of the deal – if she agreed to play along, she got to exercise some control over what they wrote.

The rest of the magazine is devoted to celebs who in one way or another are monetising their weight loss. Three have lost relatively small amounts and then become 'ambassadors' for various diet programmes. They each 'swear by' their new regime. This kind of language interests me. To swear by is to promise, to commit or to vouch for, as well as to curse. It's also a call to faith, trust and confidence. A lot of complicated emotional triggers just to recommend a diet.

Another of the celebs fronts an extremely successful line of exercise videos. She too has 'before' and 'after' photos in the same spread. Now here's a thing. It looks like they couldn't find a genuine 'before' photo for her because she's been in great shape for a long time. What they've done instead is to stretch a normal image widthways to create her 'fat before'. It's easy to spot because the whole environment – road, cars, other people – are wider than normal for their height too. This process, simple to do on any computer, produces an effect like looking in a hall of mirrors, not real, a fantasy fat version. All the better to provide contrast to the superfit 'after' photo illustrating the same article.

The message behind all these campaigns is a big old lie: 'Just do as I did and it'll be easy! And quick! Look at me, I've done it!'

But in reality it's neither simple nor speedy. And when an allegedly quick fix regime doesn't work, it makes the whole issue of weight control seem even harder than it already was, which is frankly hard enough.

When we make TV programmes we have a thing called 'compliance'. It means we have to tell the truth. If we say that they got divorced in May 2005, better make sure they did. If we say we added 50g of butter, better check that it isn't 100g. Is there no such rule governing magazines? Looking at this nonsense, I don't think so.

Magazines are also full of 'insights' that would make a grown woman weep. *Identify the emotional triggers that cause you to overeat* ... well what a stupid idea. If I could identify them they wouldn't act as triggers, would they? It's like the definition of prejudice, which is an opinion you don't recognise that you hold but that you act upon. A trigger to eat would surely be something you don't think affects you but actually sends you straight to the biscuit barrel. How could I possibly know what that might be? If I knew, I would stop it. Then it wouldn't be a trigger.

How did the diet industry become so patronising? All the material is written as if from a thin person who has never had a weight issue to an intellectually challenged child.

I have sat in WW meetings with a 'leader' holding up a carrot, asking the class to tell her what it is. 'It's a carrot.' 'Yes, but what *is* it?' This goes on for some hours (it feels like) until someone says, 'It's a vegetable!' and the leader practically screams with delight, 'That's right! That's right! You've got it!' You will of course imagine that I'm exaggerating for effect. Sadly, not so.

There is a whiff of the Puritan revivalist meeting about these encounters. 'Brothers and sisters, this woman has lost three pounds. She has seen the light. She is saved ...' Everyone claps, happy to witness virtue rewarded. If she has done well, it gives me hope. I too may be saved – by losing a pound next week.

'Not so this woman! She knows what she has done. She has sinned. She has eaten cake, she's had a whole pizza, she has had mayonnaise on chips. Woman, you know the devil is in there, let's root him out!' She is flustered, apologetic, 'Yes I know, but it was my birthday ...' or defiant, 'I don't know what happened. I was on plan the whole week. I didn't do anything wrong.' The crowd claps again, enjoying her confessional, satisfied with the promise of penance and, most of all, relieved not to be her. Is it any wonder that I prefer to sit at home alone, silently filling out an online diet tracker?

The truth is that most fat people know a great deal more about nutrition than those who have never had a weight problem. I've often been surprised by friends' questions about calories which demonstrate lack of even a basic knowledge of nutrition – and yet they're not fat. Many of us obesenics (fatties if you prefer) can name the calories in the majority of everyday food items. We know what we should eat. We just don't know how to get ourselves to actually do it.

As a student, I worked in a pub one summer and the first customer of the evening ordered a pint of beer and a bag of peanuts. Distracted, I served him, and he took out his wallet to pay.

'Five hundred and ninety-seven,' I said without thinking, quoting the number of calories in 100g bag of peanuts.

The shock on his face brought me up short. I apologised, blushing and giggling, and took his money. What this incident shows me is that all those years ago, at the age of only twenty-two, I was already completely preoccupied with calories. And has that lifelong preoccupation actually helped me to achieve or maintain a healthy weight? You already know the answer to that one.

A few years ago there was a famous case of a much-loved plump presenter who took part in an advertising campaign for a low calorie cracker. In one TV advert, she was shown, her head morphed onto a slim body, looking svelte and glam in her dressing room. An assistant appeared with a 'fat suit' consisting of her own large torso which she donned, as if it was a disguise, when called to perform. These ads were funny and self-mocking. They played with the idea that inside every fat girl is a thin girl waiting to get out. In this case, the thin girl seemed to be 'playing fat' for her job in telly. With the help of the low calorie snack, the message was that she was really thin on the inside.

What happened next was less amusing. After years in the public eye at a generous size, her weight magically dropped. She continued to advertise the product. The implication, never explicit, was that by eating it she had shed a load of weight. Then she was outed – she had had bariatric surgery. She was massively criticised for being disingenuous. She said she thought it was a private decision which she didn't need to share. So it would have been, had she not advertised the crackers. In the ensuing media furore she struck me as a forlorn and somewhat lonely figure. Before long the company had moved on and changed this marketing campaign for another.

Why does this matter? Because stories like this carry some painful messages: as if everyone knows that diet products don't really work. That in reality surgery is the only guaranteed way out of the problem. That the problem is ours alone (nothing to do with the food industry) and that we bear sole responsibility for it. Not true and not fair.

Read any magazine you care to mention and you get the impression that most adult women in the western world weigh in at around eight or nine stone and are size 8–10. And yet in the UK the average weight is nearer to eleven stone and the average dress size is 16. At five foot six I'm a little taller than the average British woman, who is apparently five foot four. For me, eleven stone is a reasonable weight but for a woman of five foot four, it's eight pounds overweight. We absorb a lot of photographic media that guides us to be a size and shape we will never be, nor even need to be. A fantasy size based on the fashion industry, or on what we used to weigh when we were twenty, or a dream of unrealisable thinness fuelled by celebrities whose income is at least partially based on their ability to stay at size zero.

Size zero, by the way, is a US size, meaning size 4–6 in the UK. But doesn't that phrase also have a ring all its own? A size so small that if you reach it, you will almost literally disappear, there will be nothing left of you. And that's the height of many women's ambitions. Not mine, I hasten to add.

Does our favourite ultra-thin heroine really live on a diet of strawberries, and not much else? Or peas alone (the single foodstuff diet)? Or frozen grapes? Articles abound that say she does, or denies that she does, or describe what she orders in restaurants, and then doesn't eat. She was decidedly chunky when she first became famous but we have seen her tripping ever more lightly through our magazine pages over the years, and watched her transform herself gradually into an elegant wraith. Her current slenderness is fascinating and troubling at the same time. There's an air of fragility about her which doesn't look like self-care or relaxation, but massive self-restraint bordering on self-deprivation. It's her choice, of course, but she's a role model for thousands of young women who will struggle to mimic her 'achievement' in being so thin.

I would love to imagine a world where being healthy and comfortable was celebrated. How is it that actor A and presenter B have to tolerate articles about their 'generous' figures? Generous? Give me strength. They're both beautiful young women who are nowhere near overweight, let alone obese, and yet their body size is continually held up to comment and criticism. With that sort of nonsense swilling around the media, it's no wonder that so many of us are self-critical and anguished about our bodies because we can't reach that elusive, ever-desired incredible lightness of being.

It seems there is no space for middle-sized. We are teetering on anorexia, desperately craving unachievable thinness, or else obsessing about being overweight, gathering pounds and angst hand in hand.

Having said that, of course, none of the above really applies to me. I'm not just self-critical without reason. I actually am clinically obese. I was nearly morbidly obese. I've pulled back from the brink. There's a pleasure in writing these sentences, because they are factual. They sound self-flagellating, but that's because in our culture we are so emotionally charged about this whole subject. In fact 'I am obese' is not self-judgement, but simply an accurate description since my BMI is over 30. Now at BMI 37, down by 2.4 points from where I began. Still going down.

The language of obesity categories is telling. The word 'obesity' comes from the Latin meaning 'having eaten until fat' and 'morbid' means diseased. There's severe, morbid, super morbid and extreme obesity. They all refer to specific numbers of BMI points but they have a ring of judgement about them. It's no surprise that in America these loaded phrases are being replaced by obesity classes 1–3, satisfyingly clinical descriptors, where Class 3 is BMI 40+. Introducing numbered classes has an added benefit: it makes it very easy to add more categories should need demand. Sad to say, at the rate we're going, need will demand.

The problem for the western world is that average weights are rising. Over half of us are now tipping into the obese category.

Yet as we get fatter, we are constantly absorbing images of unrealistic thinness. Is it just me, or is this completely crazy?

However, indignation about this state of affairs doesn't mean that I shouldn't lose my own excess and get to a healthy weight. To some people that will sound obvious, but I'm sorry to say that for me it's worth a reminder.

My own ambitions are modest. I picture myself in a crowd on a London street. Someone scans the view and is asked to describe it. Their eyes do not stop at me. They do not say, 'There was a plump woman in a grey coat by the bus stop' or 'Oh yes, the fat woman – she wore a red skirt'. They don't notice me, because I have a BMI of 25, and am unremarkable among the rest.

It's a distant dream.

I AM A detective, looking for clues, causes and motivations.

As a toddler I was a little rounded but at the normal end of the spectrum. By the age of eight I was already a seasoned dieter. The first, at six, was nothing to do with obesity but followed an operation to remove my tonsils. For weeks afterwards my throat was so painful that any solid food felt like sandpaper. I lived on liquids, mostly soup and mashed banana, until it healed. I remember the savoury smell of sausages frying for breakfast which I couldn't eat.

I don't know what happened, but over the next year or two, the various adults in my life began putting me on a series of diets. There was a particularly ironic twist to this.

My parents separated just before my tonsil operation and both found new partners. We children were offered the choice of which one we wanted to live with. Unlike my siblings, I kept changing my mind, too young to fully commit to one over the other and desperately missing whoever I was separated from. I remember the pain of having to break it to each in turn that I wanted to move again. And although, looking back, it seems totally crazy that they let me keep swapping, for them it was a matter of principle to give us that terrible choice and they stuck by it. The result is that I was an eleven by eleven: by the age of eleven, I'd been to eleven schools. As already noted, I also weighed eleven stone.

Here's the irony. When I was in Cornwall with my father and kind-of stepmother, the family naturally fell into two groups. Two of my older brothers and my middle sister were still at home but old enough to be either at work or secondary school, and so they ate with the adults. From being the youngest of my mother's children, I had morphed into the eldest of the little kids, my stepmother's four children, who ranged in age from one to five. She nominated me their unofficial nursemaid and, aged seven, it was my job to cook for them each evening while she and my father prepared the adult supper. I made us scrambled eggs or beans on toast, spaghetti hoops or pasta. I don't remember my feelings about this task but it was a big (food-related) responsibility to be given very young.

My mother was kinder in many ways, but now that I examine it strangely similar in others. She was based in London by then and had trained, late in life, as a chef. When I next went to live with her, she was cooking in a fancy West End restaurant where she had designed a 1960s-style luxury menu – avocados with prawn cocktail, beef stroganoff and charlotte russe. These foods felt like a touch of the high life and I loved them.

Working in a commercial kitchen is physically gruelling and the last thing my mother wanted to do when she came home was to cook, so she paid me a pound a week to do the housekeeping. It meant shopping and cooking for her, my twelve-year-old brother Crispin and myself. She earned £14 per week as a head chef in 1964, which means my 'wages' for this work were worth about £50 per week at today's values.

In dire contrast to the food she was serving at the restaurant, I fed us gourmet à la nine-year-old: Fray Bentos steak and kidney pies, tinned new potatoes and peas. Or shepherd's pie made with tinned mince and Smash instant mashed potato.

My other favourites were Vesta ready meals. They were the first Indian and Chinese foods available to cook at home in this country. Each box held a series of little packets – rice, poppadums and mango chutney with the curry or crispy fried noodles, prawn crackers and egg fried rice with the chow mein. I knew they were of questionable quality but they were easy to make and even from my child's perspective, a great guilty pleasure. And I loved the little packets.

So both my mother and my stepmother relied on me, as a young child, to cook for them every day. A heavy load when I should have been playing hopscotch. My brother and sister used to call me 'Wee Slavey' after the cartoon strip in the girls' comic *Judy*. The heroine was a child servant called Nellie in a Victorian household. Although put-upon, Nellie was smart and clever so at the time I quite liked this nickname. In retrospect it has a different ring.

I must have ballooned at this time, I suppose, because both my mother and stepmother separately took me to task for putting on weight and put me on various restrictive diets to help me lose it. Only it didn't feel like helping. It felt like criticism.

Luckily, I've always loved cooking and these early experiences didn't stifle that. Perhaps they even fostered it – there's only so much Smash you can make before you realise that peeling a potato and steaming it yourself makes for a better result. I mull on this while I rustle up coleslaw with vinaigrette for tonight's supper. Large piles of raw, plant-based food with a few nuts thrown in for protein. Utterly virtuous, utterly delicious.

*

FOR MANY YEARS, I believed that it isn't possible to force yourself to diet when you're not ready. However much you want to, you can't 'pull yourself together', even though that's what your own inner critic keeps telling you to do.

Every now and then a light would come on and I would get into the zone for a bit. I would grab those opportunities eagerly and make the best of them while I could. But they were often short lived and when gone, I was exasperatingly unable to find the courage and motivation to start again.

Is this really how it has to be? Do you have to wait for a moment of inspiration to descend like a ray of sunshine streaking through the clouds – which allows you to do it? I'm beginning to doubt the truth of that. I have a glimmer of an idea that you can prepare yourself mentally, and then begin.

I draw up a list of 'last straws' that got me going this time:

1. My hands becoming so pudgy that I couldn't wear my wedding and engagement rings for over a year. Finally, a couple of months ago, I got them altered. It was tricky and expensive, because it took extra gold to make them big enough. I'm wearing them now, but every time I look at them I think, 'This is ridiculous.'
2. Photographs taken at our Christmas lunch last year – me as Mrs Potato Head in a yellow paper hat and a loud rosy shirt. And a face of shocked plump misery.
3. Buying a new bra – size 42H. Not funny.
4. Tipping over seventeen stone for the only time in my life apart from when I was nine months pregnant.
5. Asking myself which would I prefer – to win the lottery or lose six stone. The answer sprung immediately to mind: I would lose the weight. And in a heartbeat I realised that that was something I actually have the power to do, whereas of course I can't do anything to affect whether I win the lottery beyond buying the ticket.
6. Imagining I had a terrible illness – cancer, diabetes, a stroke. Knowing that if that happened I would immediately change my lifestyle and my eating habits. Why wait till I get ill? Decide to pretend that I've had the diagnosis already, and act accordingly.

7. Making a cookery series with a rugby legend-turned-chef presenter. At dinner on the road, I notice how he eats. He orders steak and chips, but never has more than a couple of the chips, none of the fat on the steak, never pudding. No chocolate or biscuits during the shoot, which everyone else snacks on to keep them going. I watch and learn. He makes no fuss about this and I can see it's not an effort, just a lifestyle decision.

Just a lifestyle decision. Sounds so easy, doesn't it? How do you talk yourself into making new lifestyle decisions when you've made the wrong ones by mistake?

This becomes my new mantra: Just a lifestyle decision. Just a lifestyle decision. No biggie. Just a lifestyle decision.

Sobering fact #6: *The global weight loss industry was worth $176 billion in 2017. And yet obesity rates continue to rise.*

Research and Markets, 2017

CHAPTER 7

Who is Bridget? What is she?

16st 3lb

Saturday, 30 July 2011

It's sunrise on the tor, an orange streak above a charcoal landscape. It's going to be a hot day, but for now the air is still and sharp. Only the clatter of the waking birds breaks the silence.

Bridget is busy. She's trundling a wheelbarrow full of wood and cut sods of earth across the moorland. Her hair, in a thick wispy plait, falls over one shoulder, and bounces as she wheels her load from the woods to her cave.

'Hi,' I call to her.

She nods curtly.

'I just came to say thanks.' It's a bit embarrassing, having to thank someone who doesn't speak to you. I'm afraid she'll find me gushy.

She looks straight at me, and then carries on with her work. I can see she's listening. That's encouragement enough to plough on.

'It seems to be going well. My diet. I'm managing to stick to it … I'm losing weight.' Again that sensation that I'm stuttering, nervous in the face of her impassivity.

It feels like talking to a deaf person who refuses to turn on their hearing aid. But she's obviously not hearing-impaired, just not very interested.

'OK then. Thought you'd like to know.'

She grins, kindly, distracted, throws her untidy plait over her shoulder and carries on trundling.

A TRICKY WEEK with two very tough shoot days, but I still managed to shift a pound. Only one more to go till I've lost my first stone. I feel very different but few people have even noticed. That's fine – it's still a private enterprise for now.

Buoyed by my little bit of success, I burble to Chris about the challenges and the progress of my diet, but he's fairly unresponsive. He has never been seriously overweight himself and so doesn't know much about the technicalities of calorie control. Lucky him.

I'm on a generous allowance of thirty-three WW points per day plus a weekly allowance of forty-nine extra WW points. That's roughly equivalent to 1800 calories per day plus as much fruit and vegetables as I can eat. Plenty. As far as hunger is concerned, it's really not hard to stick to this.

I am committed to telling the truth about this journey and something troubles me. This is the truth, but it's far from the whole truth. Despite appearances, and all that I've written so far, my life is not and has not been dominated by food. Being a wife and mother, relationships with family and friends, and a huge enthusiasm for my work are all much more important. But like white noise disturbing the atmosphere, annoying, upsetting and distracting, anxieties about what I've eaten and how much I weigh have been in the background all the time. For now, I'm concentrating on that white noise, and trying to see it off. I'm logging this because I would hate you to think that this food thing is all there is to me. It's just the bit that I need to work on right now.

An enthusiastic cook myself, as already mentioned, I also produce food programmes. I can almost hear you say, 'Oh well, there you are then. That's where your problem lies.'

But I don't think that's true at all. For me, cooking for my family and friends, and myself, being interested in provenance and enjoying dishes from around the world are all the healthy aspects of my relationship with food.

Unfortunately, alongside those bits I have a problem, which is mild, consistent overeating. You might not think that if you had dinner with me when my consumption probably wouldn't strike you (or me) as excessive. The proof is in the numbers. My weight has climbed seven stone in the forty years since I was a student.

It's only two and a half pounds per year.

That's all it takes to end up here.

BY THE AGE of ten I felt like a blimp, round face, round tummy, chubby thighs. I had developed a passion for Lyons fruit pies, apple or apricot, sixpence a go from vending machines at most railway stations up and down the land. I spent a lot of time on my own at railway stations, travelling between Cornwall and London, father and mother. The pies were crisp and round with a glittering sugar-encrusted top. When you bit into them they contained mostly air, a thin layer of semi-pureed fruit sitting on the base, cavernous emptiness above. As with most fast food, the pleasure was fleeting but the calories were not.

Late one night while I was staying in London with my mother, a call came to tell us that my father had died. He had been ill with cancer for months but I had had no idea how serious it was. I was in shock for weeks, blank-faced and grim, desperate to go to his funeral but forbidden to. My mother couldn't bear to meet my stepmother there so decided not to go herself. Without her, no one wanted to take responsibility for yet another young child at this stressful time. Up until then, I had been treated as a quasi-adult, responsible for the younger ones, their cook and keeper. Now that tragedy struck, I was suddenly relegated to child status again and discussed as though I was a little kid. It was very confusing.

After his death, time disappeared for a while. I lost about six months from my memory. Always chaotic, my mother's emotional life unravelled and she tumbled from one unsatisfactory relationship to another. Our fractured family, consisting of two constantly shifting households, was split in half. From then on, I rarely saw my younger half siblings until adulthood.

Meanwhile my mother sent me to an inner city comprehensive school for a term or so, although I was barely ten, too young to be there. This was Risinghill, a famously semi-progressive school due for closure by the local authority because its teaching methods were so contentious. Specifically, they disapproved of the fact that the head had banned the use of the cane, which was considered a dangerously liberal strategy. When Risinghill closed, the education department insisted that I return to a junior school for two more terms. I was sent to Hampstead Primary, a privileged and solidly middle-class school tucked in an alleyway behind Hampstead Tube.

Dazed and distracted, I was used to learning on the hoof, having to pick up lessons halfway through a term or syllabus, only half understanding most of what was going on around me. To my astonishment, when I left at the end of that summer term I was given a pencil case with a card saying I had completed my final year 'With Distinction'. It was the first time I had ever done well academically. I ran home, airy lightness coursing through my veins, lifting me six inches above the pavement all the way.

My eldest sister, Julia, by now married with two small children, then threw me a lifeline. She realised that all this ricocheting from school to school was hopeless for me. She took me to live with her and found an independent girls' school nearby which I could go to. My mother agreed readily enough. Her dramatic relationships were probably easier to handle without a child in tow.

It was a sharp contrast to the life I had led till then and to all the many schools I had dipped into and out of. My education had included a nearly full house of every type of school on offer in England at that time. There were progressive schools, church schools, inner city schools, village schools and fancy private schools, poor schools and rich schools, liberal schools and rigid schools. The only card missing from the pack was a boarding school.

Sunny Hill combined day, weekly boarding and full boarding options and had grammar school places too. The private pupils came mostly from forces families and the grammar pupils were farmers' daughters drawn from the surrounding area. This mixed culture suited me and I stayed for the full seven years of my secondary schooling, sometimes boarding and sometimes not. I've been grateful to my sister ever since for finding it, persuading everyone that it was the best course for me and making it happen.

In my first year at this new school, my class was picked to do a dance on speech day based on Oscar Wilde's story 'The Selfish Giant'. I was cast as the giant. My classmates played cute children tumbling in my orchard and I had to stomp in and scare them all away.

I felt that I had been singled out to look ridiculous and I hated it. In fact I was so mortified that a few days before the performance I decided to pretend I'd sprained my ankle. I had to beg hard to get Julia to back me up. She was worried that I would regret giving up the role, but when she understood that the idea of performing was causing me real agony, she gamely played along.

The understudy was a girl called Marian Gaskell who loved the limelight and was delighted to step in. I still remember the smell of warm damp cut grass and the summer haze as I looked down onto the terrace where Marian performed, clomping around in a big red velvet doublet and hose. I sat nursing my bandaged ankle with relief. I would have had to wear those horrors. To my astonishment, Marian seemed to be enjoying herself. It was many years before I looked back and realised that I had been given the lead role in that dance, and had rejected it.

Contact with my mother for the next few years was restricted to her sudden, startling swoops into the Somerset countryside. She would descend like Zeus from Mount Olympus, bearing gifts and telling stories. By then she worked for a catering agency and she was posted to hotels and country houses all over Britain who were in need of a chef for a short time to cover illness, or cook for parties or events. Her tales of work were full of angels and demons, those she loved and those she loathed. Only extremes were worth the telling.

Between these visits I would call her, reversing the charges, standing on one foot in the chilly red phone box on the village green, keeping her talking because I missed her. 'Darling, I must rush ...' was her usual sign off.

TWO OF THE clichés about obesity are that it's either a kind of self-punishment or leads to self-disgust. They are not the same thing but are related ideas. I'm not sure that either is true for me. My self-confidence has always been based on things other than my physical self – being emotionally in touch, working hard and creatively, being reliable and strong. I used to tell myself that I just wasn't vain enough to care what I looked like. It was comforting, and chimed with my feminist sensibilities, almost as though I had made a positive choice not to pay attention to my body. But it rang a little hollow, too. I didn't quite believe it myself. I wanted to, but I couldn't.

Being fat is uncomfortable. Clothes don't hang well. Knickers and tights pinch. Changing rooms are torture chambers. Where on earth did the stereotype of the jolly fat person come from? Being fat is not jolly. I was always hungry too, and yet constantly fighting the desire to eat the wrong things. Ironically, it's much easier to enjoy food as well as to feel full when you consume it more judiciously.

When I met Chris I weighed just over twelve stone. By the time we married, three years later, I was 13st 8lb. I had dieted for the wedding but only managed to chisel off a few pounds and, afterwards, in the happiness and relaxation of a new relationship, my weight gradually increased. Every few months, Chris would try to talk me into dieting for the sake of my health. For him, it was a source of deep fear. He imagined that I would become disabled, dependent, or even die young because of obesity. I thought he was being ridiculous.

Chris's father, Elwyn, spent most of his life at around twenty-three stone. He was six foot six, a huge rumbling Welshman, a wonderful storyteller with great personality, and he carried his vast bulk off with such aplomb that it wasn't the first or even the second thing that would occur to you if you were to describe him. But, like my mother, in his sixties he developed diabetes.

He didn't trouble to find out much about it. He decided that he might be prone to hypoglycaemia and, just in case of an attack, kept a Mars bars in his glove compartment at all times. By the end of each day, when he hadn't needed it to stave off the putative hypo, he would eat it anyway and then replace it, only to repeat the whole sequence the next day. In reality of course he was doing the exact opposite of what was needed to control his diabetes. It's very rare indeed for Type 2 diabetics to suffer from hypos and, as far as I'm aware, he never had one. The most effective treatment would have been a low calorie diet coupled with exercise to curb the obesity which had almost certainly led to the disease in the first place.

Unlike my mother, Elwyn died very suddenly of a heart attack, aged sixty-seven. This was only a few years after Chris and I married. Chris was deeply shocked. He had always realised his dad was heavy but for some reason it had never occurred to him that he might die young. It affected Chris profoundly and motivated him to turn his attention to his own weight and fitness, which began to improve dramatically. Like his father he is tall, but unlike him, Chris has always been a healthy weight for his six foot four height. But he was very conscious of a tendency to put on the pounds around his middle, the area sometimes known as heart attack fat. He looked at what had happened to his dad and felt his path was absolutely clear. He began to run and cycle two or three times a week and to watch what he ate.

From my perspective, he became somewhat preoccupied with ageing, disease and early death. This will come as news to his friends who know him as funny, easy-going and, in that familiar old phrase, 'so laid back he's almost horizontal', as one of them said to me recently. She was surprised when I raised an eyebrow. 'Up to a point,' I said.

His new outlook was fine, if a little morose, until he began to turn his attention to me. He would keep quiet for months and then, usually late at night, lying in bed just before sleep, he would raise the subject. For him it was simple. His much-loved father and my mother (whom he never met) had both died younger than they should have done as a direct result of obesity. He couldn't understand why this knowledge didn't motivate me to lose weight. He called it cognitive dissonance, which I thought frankly rude.

These discussions never ended well. I would become defensive and would explain at length why I simply couldn't lose weight, how busy and tired I was, how the metabolism slows down in middle age, making it virtually impossible for me to succeed, how I kept trying to diet and it didn't work. The talking would escalate quickly into a row. I would get angry and tearful, and feel as if he was threatening to leave me. He said it was the other way round – that I would leave him by dying young when there was no need for it. He would be much more reasonable than me but insistent, persuasive and unbending. I would promise to try another diet, really would try and do my best. I would cry some more. These conversations were very painful for both of us. They happened every few months over the next fifteen years.

Was it cognitive dissonance? Meaning that I was holding two contradictory ideas and feeling uncomfortable because they clashed? Well yes. I knew my eating habits were unhealthy and yet I continued to overeat. I also didn't enjoy being fat, and yet I still overate. The discomfort arose from protecting my own position: yes, I know it's very bad for me, but I feel literally unable to do anything about it. Instead of admitting to that sense of impotence, I would drum up copious reasons why it was actually impossible. Fear and despair ruled. So yes, it was cognitive dissonance.

One year he tried to make me promise to lose weight by a certain age. 'A BMI of 25 by the time you're fifty-two,' he said. But how could I possibly agree to that when I felt completely unable to do it? If I would be able to do it when I was fifty-two, then I could do it now. I couldn't. If I couldn't do it now, why was I going to be able to by the time I was fifty-two?

It reminded me of when I was in labour, my spinal fluid flooded with anaesthetic, and then they told me to push. You might as well have asked me to push down the wall of the delivery room by sheer effort of will. I couldn't do it, and couldn't see how I ever would.

Another year at Christmas I gave him, among other presents, a stone. It was supposed to represent a stone I was committing to lose. A foolish promise, impossible to keep. He looked sceptical – rightly, as it turned out. I shed a few pounds and then stalled again.

TODAY CHRIS HAS given me a book which is already, only a few pages in, mind-blowing. *Thinking, Fast and Slow* describes how our thought processes are not linear, but are driven by what psychologist Daniel Kahneman calls two systems. 'System 1' is associative, cumulative, perceptive of change and alert for danger, while 'system 2' is verbal, rational, reasoning and takes care of planning ahead.

Over years of research he has shown that 'system 1' is the brain's first response. It's quick and automatic, designed to maintain the status quo and is not reflective, but protects us from harm by constantly scanning for danger. 'System 2' is more considered, more capable of change, but slow. It is also very energy consuming and, he says, lazy. It doesn't want to do the work. So where it can, the brain takes the line of least resistance and leaves instant decision-making to 'system 1'.

I keep reading late into the night, utterly absorbed. From those early delvings into Freud and Jung, read years ago, my picture of the unconscious was of a hidden part of the personality, dark and dangerous territory, the source of surreal dreams, animal instincts and unexpressed desires. Benjamin Libet, on the other hand, didn't interpret the unconscious, or speculate on its motives, so much as show that it exists and is active. At first my understanding was so programmed by Freud's narrative that I assumed Kahneman's 'system 1' was equivalent to his theory of the unconscious. But Kahneman doesn't claim that 'system 1' is unconscious, just that it's a fast worker. Gradually I began to see that he has developed an entirely new theory of mind.

Through careful, intelligent experiments he shows how we think in different ways and at different speeds according to the task set and the circumstances. He also shows how 'system 1', calling on its vast collection of associative memories, can be misled into making poor decisions – prejudiced, confused or simply mistaken – which 'system 2' will usually rush to back up and post-rationalise. That's the real kicker. 'System 2' is better at absorbing new information and ideas and making rational judgements, but out of idleness it prefers not to do the work. It's easier to support the prejudices of 'system 1' instead.

He shows that we are complex, inconsistent and, contrary to previous economic theory, neither entirely selfish nor totally altruistic. It's compelling reading.

MY FIRST THOUGHT is that Bridget is the embodiment of Daniel Kahneman's 'system 1'. In my imagination, when it comes to making decisions, she calls the shots. I feel like her supplicant. She is non-verbal but ultimately powerful. She doesn't articulate her choices but they are clear – she votes with her feet. What she wants is what I do.

Instead I could say 'I do what she wants' but that would suggest I know what she wants and I don't, because she doesn't verbalise. In fact, it's only by observing my own actions that I have any clue what she's up to.

The rules for this game unrolled themselves when I first dreamed her up. Bridget is not talkative, of course, and she can't be charmed or brought round by flattery. Like an animal, she responds to body language, pictures and gestures more than to words. At the time, I recognised that there were unconscious mechanisms spurring me on to addictive behaviour around food. However much I tried to grasp why, whatever I thought I had come to understand, did not in the end affect my behaviour or help me to alter it.

What I hoped to do by inventing Bridget was to re-programme my own thinking.

Deep in the book, I feel called to her presence.

<hr />

'What do you want?' I ask.

A ball of wool is in a muddle around her feet. She seems distracted. I pick it up and start to wind it up for her. She smiles, vague but not displeased.

I sense that she perceives herself as ultimately alone. She thinks she needs no one, huddling round a rough brazier at twilight in her cave. She appears so emotionally remote that it's hard to believe she's even connected to me, but of course she is. It would be a grave mistake to underestimate her power.

'Do you enjoy my visits?'

She shrugs like an awkward teenager.

My only way forward is to respect her and cherish her. She is me, but she's also in control of me. When this gets really tough it's Bridget I turn to, although she never turns to me.

'I hope to find out more as time goes by.' I hand back a neatly wound ball of wool, the end tucked in.

She picks at it with one bony finger. She doesn't answer.

As usual, I don't really know if she's listened to anything I say, but the proof seems to be in the pudding. She's allowing me to make healthy choices. She's giving me a sense of longed-for control and I'm grateful for that.

'Good to see you.' I wave goodbye, as if to a friend, and really begin to feel that we could get on.

COULD IT BE that she's not just a strange stray figment of my imagination, but that she represents a real psychological phenomenon? The parallels with 'system 1' are striking and exciting.

Is that why I seem to be making changes where I never could before? I'm two months into this diet, and feel stuck in. I committed to a year with no real sense that I could keep to it, but now it seems as though I can. I'm elated.

Be careful what you wish for. I found a wise woman who's a bit of a witch. She means well by me, I'm sure, but I wish she was less witchy.

Sobering fact #7: *More men are overweight or obese than women. In 2015, 68 per cent of men in the UK were overweight or obese compared with 58 per cent of women.*

House of Commons Library, 2017

CHAPTER 8

This is not a proper diet book

16st 1lb

Saturday, 13 August 2011

'Bridget – I'm going on holiday.'

I've come to know that look. It seems to say, 'Statement of the bleeding obvious mate!'

She sits swinging her legs over the edge of a gigantic rock, for once not busy. Maybe she's on holiday too.

'I just want to say – I could do with some help while I'm away. I don't want to undo all the good I've done.'

She throws her head back, gazing at the sky. She doesn't glance in my direction. She might as well have said, 'Well, don't.'

'"Well, don't?" Is that as profound as it gets?'

She nods curtly. I stomp back down the hill. I'd been hoping for some strength to keep myself on track. But as I clamber down, I begin to see her point. It really is as simple as that. Well, don't.

I'M ASTONISHED TO find that I do not have tiny pinprick eyes. I've lost just over a stone now, and it's really beginning to show. The real shock is my face. It had honestly never occurred to me that my eyes were small because they were lost in a pad of fat. I feel very stupid when I look at them now – they're beginning to emerge from the folds. This is so much cheaper and safer than surgery.

Writing this diary began as a personal project to help me unravel the tangle of ideas in my head about my obesity. But now it's underway, and my stumbling methods have astonishingly started to work, I wonder if other people might get something from it too. But what is it? Not a proper diet book: there are no unrealistic goals, no immediate solutions, no huge promises of sudden transformation at the end. I only mention what I eat in passing, in case anyone is interested, but I'm assuming they will know all about calories, exercise and making good food choices. I'm assuming that like me, they know all that but don't or can't act on it.

Perhaps the best way to look at this journal is as a companion to a diet, any diet. What I really want to share is the story of how I am rethinking the whole issue. It's taken me fifty years to get here. For me it's been very slow.

It's the story of a long and arduous struggle. You could say it began when I was nine years old and first began to get chubby. I've been on and off diets ever since. You could say it started on 4 June 2011, when I signed up to Weight Watchers this time. Or you could date it from an excruciating conversation that took place two years before that, after Cadover Bridge, after Benjamin Libet, but before I had worked out what to do with those revelations.

At breakfast one morning Chris and I stumbled into a conversation about my weight. He had obviously been working up to one of his regular assaults on the subject but it was unusual for it to happen over breakfast. I hadn't seen it coming, and was shocked and unresponsive.

He tells me now that he was desperate and didn't know how to motivate me to change. He launched what felt like a full-scale attack. He said I was like an alcoholic, unable to give up over-eating, addicted despite what I knew it was likely to do to my health. I understood the analogy. My family has had its share of alcoholics and I know first-hand what that means. It made me absolutely furious.

'What, do I eat the family income – or earn it? Do I cause emotional and financial chaos all around me – or help to support us all? Do I sacrifice everyone and everything so that I can have just one more baked potato – or cook for everyone? Do I empty our kid's money box to buy chocolate? What are you talking about?' And so on.

He sat up, energised. 'There you are. You'll do anything to defend your position. Look at how angry you are.'

There's nothing more infuriating than being told you're angry when you actually are very angry. You can't deny it, and to admit it feels like giving ground.

I listened to him explaining – again – how dangerous he thought it was for me to be so heavy, and something in me rebelled. I was sick of being nagged and being made to feel rubbish on a regular basis. I've always told him that he shouldn't go into coaching as a profession. In a situation like this he is the opposite of encouraging, not so much a cheerleader as a doomsayer. For once I got mulish and set my face against him. No more 'Yes I do see, I really do realise, I'll try, give me time, I'll get going tomorrow.'

I said I just couldn't do it, couldn't lose. I said that it's harder for everyone to control weight in middle age (really? Is that true, or a cop out?).

That it was actually almost impossible because the fat had accumulated over such a long period that it was now a fixture (not true).

That it was pointless to say I would because I knew I couldn't (not true).

I said, 'I'm tired of promising you that I will, only to find that I won't. It makes a fool of me, and it doesn't give you what you want.'

This is the only bit of all the above that still has a real ring of truth about it, by the way. This bit was the truth as I saw it then, among a lot of nonsense.

Finally I asked, 'So what will happen if I don't?'

Without hesitation he replied, 'I might just run off with a thin bint.'

'Now you've said something really destructive.' I didn't recognise my own voice.

I cried and couldn't stop, tears spurting from my eyes, splashing onto my hands. I couldn't go to work (unheard of), couldn't stop sobbing, was bereft. Couldn't see how I was going to forgive him for threatening to leave me, actually naming what I feared most.

He was kind. He patted me, and kept telling me it would be alright. It seemed to me he was waiting for the usual capitulation – yes I do see, I really will try, etc. But I wasn't willing to offer it because I had finally recognised how untruthful it would be. He was immediately contrite about the 'thin bint' remark and claimed that he had made it to shock me into action. I'm not sure I buy that. It was a very quick response: a bit 'system 1', if you get my drift.

He was trying to comfort me but something had shifted. He kept saying, 'It's OK, I love you, we'll get through this.'

But I wasn't so sure that we would. I felt I couldn't bear to have that same conversation with him ever again. Every time it happened it was agonising and demotivating and just succeeded in making me feel a failure. I've achieved a few things in other areas of my life, but in this particular department it's been a struggle all the way.

The next day I was back at work, trying to push this conflict to the back of my mind. It was difficult but I managed to get through the day somehow. Driving back across the moor, listening to music in the car, I thought ruefully about going home. It's always felt like returning to the fold, to warmth, love and comfort. But not this time. I dreaded returning to the same ongoing row.

I knew that Chris and I would be united in keeping it from Orlando, but I was far from over it. Chris himself was still loving and reassuring, as if to forgive me. But to be honest he seemed rather too secure of me, confident that my love for him would overcome this. I wasn't in the same place. I felt that this time he had gone too far.

Just as I was steeling myself for the evening ahead, the radio started to play a track by The Nylons. 'You're the one I turn to, No one cares like you do.'

I welled up. My marriage had always seemed unassailable but now was shaken to the core by this stupid row about my weight. I really didn't think I could forgive Chris for the thin bint remark. He is normally the person I rely on in times of worry and distress, but now was the very person I couldn't turn to. Then what? Separation? Divorce? As I drove into our garage, instead of the usual joyful homecoming I was filled with fear.

He was taken aback. He thought we'd moved on and were getting over it. Instead he had a weepy wife, a mess in an overcoat, stumbling through the door, stricken.

One of the strengths of our relationship is that we both like a rational argument. I think that's what saved us. In a good marriage, when you disagree, it's sometimes (not always) really hard to work out who is right. You love the other person and trust their judgement and yet it's clashing with your own. This was one of those knotty wrangles and we had to thrash it out.

Over the next few weeks we took long walks across Dartmoor in the drizzle, the dog leaping around us as though nothing was wrong. Chris painted a picture of my future, sick, dependent on him (and he thought he'd make a terrible nurse), getting less and less mobile while he was getting fitter, our lives moving apart, and eventually me dying young. He had it all mapped out in his mind. I swallowed my irritation and listened. I pointed out that it could just as easily be him that ended up disabled and dependent – fit people get struck down too. Yes, he said, but statistically you're loading the dice against yourself. There was no arguing with that.

I told him about my sense of powerlessness. I explained that every time I told myself I was going to diet, I would find within minutes that I was eating something disastrous, as though I had no independent motor function. The crazy thing was that it was never a huge amount of food – I've never been a binger. But a daily supermarket meal deal for lunch and a nightly bag of crisps or bar of chocolate on the way home while shopping for supper, along with regular bad menu choices, was enough to gradually creep on the pounds, and ultimately the stones.

We talked and talked. Eventually I proposed a compromise of sorts. I said that I couldn't stand him badgering me about my weight problem anymore. I wanted it to be a no go area. In return, I would take responsibility for it. His restraint wouldn't let me off the hook from having to do something about it. We would each have something to give up: him, the right to lecture, and me, inaction.

I could tell that he considered this a pretty weak offer, but I meant it. It took me another two years of thinking about it, taking a run up at it, worrying about it, but at last I'm keeping my side of the bargain.

At the time, Chris didn't like it. He said he felt silenced. He said he raised these issues with me 'for your own good' and he couldn't deal with not being allowed to talk about it. I was resolute. I said I was sorry that he felt that way but that it was how it had to be. I wouldn't be shamed into accepting that kind of talk any more. I felt powerless to change, but the one thing I was sure of was that those late-night interventions were not productive. I don't know what suddenly gave me that certainty after so many years, but something did.

CHRIS LOOKS OVER my shoulder and reads what I've written so far. He wants to have his say (so go write your own book!). He describes those years as anxious, fearing that I would either die young or become incapacitated like my mother, dependent on carers and family to function. He would keep quiet as long as he could and then feel he must bring it to my attention. He felt he was doing it for my benefit and finds it painful to hear how it was for me.

Two more years after the rings that wouldn't fit, more private anxieties and the final stone on the weighing scales. And here I am.

So when I started this diet, you can see why I didn't want to involve him. I had told him that he couldn't talk about my weight so I could hardly raise it with him. And anyway, I had set off on this particular jaunt so many times before – why was this time going to be different?

I still don't really know what's changed. Perhaps it helped that, from the start, mentally, I signed up for a year. That means I was at least trying to be realistic about the timescale. Or it could be learning mindfulness – that's certainly been a big step forward.

My real instinct, though, is that the most powerful weapon in my armoury is Bridget. She's been the key to recognising the role of the unconscious. She is a way of dealing with it. If I remember to think about her, I stay on track. When I forget to, I stray. I invented her as a way of training my mind to act in harmony with itself. I had no idea how well it would work. It's been a revelation.

WE'RE ON HOLIDAY, gliding up the Nile on a cruiser. The biggest challenge for me is a lavish hotel breakfast followed by two four-course meals a day. There's afternoon tea too, if we should be struck by sudden hunger mid-afternoon. I avoid bread and choose lighter options from the menu. It's the height of summer, boiling, mid-Ramadan and mid-revolution. Hardly the ideal time for our visit, but we love it. We lap up the history of the pyramids and the temples along every mile of the river. Egypt's influence on Art Deco is obvious everywhere I look, spurred by the discovery in 1922 of Tutankhamun's tomb – lotus, papyrus and scarab; dark earthy reds, rich blues, deep greens and gold.

There are only eight guests on a boat built for a hundred so we get to know each other quite well. Brad, a young, fit American fellow traveller orders eggs for breakfast every morning but eats only the whites. Even at twenty-four, slim and fit, he is weight conscious. In a country where poverty is rife, throwing away the yolks seems a little tasteless but, to be fair, when he's my age he won't be fat.

At the end of our trip, to my amazement and delight, I've stayed the same weight. It's a triumph. Chris isn't surprised, but I am. He had noticed me peel batter off fish and discard it, choose salad not carbs, fruit not pudding. He saw that I was focused and he was optimistic on my behalf. For my part, I had tried not to undo all the good of the last few months without much belief that my efforts at damage limitation would actually work, but they did. I realised that I have come to think of weight gain as almost inevitable, unavoidable, a crocodile pit waiting for me to fall in. Turns out that's wrong. In fact, it's possible to take control and that's exactly what I had done.

This is a pivotal moment. Sixteen stone and what do you get? Another day older and deeper in fret. That's OK because I'm leaving sixteen stone behind me, never going back again.

Sobering fact #8: *'Weight watching' is by no means female territory anymore – 65 per cent of women and 44 per cent of men in Britain tried to lose weight in 2013.*

Mintel, 2014

CHAPTER 9

Snap, crackle and pop

15st 10lb

Saturday, 10 September 2011

Bridget is making her way across a patch of quaking bog, like quicksand, on the moor. I watch her, heart in mouth in case she slips, but she's sure-footed.

I know from local folklore that if you fall the best thing you can do is to stretch out like a starfish and wait until rescue comes. It slows down the rate of getting sucked in.

'Wait for me,' I call.

She glances back but doesn't noticeably slow up.

'Where are we going?' No answer.

'Do you want me to follow you?' No answer.

I struggle to keep up, avoiding pitfalls as I go. I wish she'd talk to me.

This is what you call one-way communication.

What do I do if I trip? Lie spread-eagled and wait for rescue? Don't think so. I'll swim out backstroke if I have to.

FIVE POUNDS LOST in four weeks. Steady progress.

Lying in bed, listening to my body fizzing and popping with change, I can actually feel myself losing weight, like a bowl of breakfast cereal snapping and crackling. I run my hands over my torso, trying to get used to its new shape, feeling for differences. My hip bones are emerging after years hidden in folds of fat.

I have no idea what size I am any more. If there's a gap behind someone's chair I can't estimate whether I'll fit if I slide through. It's disconcerting, but in a good way.

This week I was inspired by the sight of Marianne, glimpsed across the room at a party. She's someone I know in passing, a familiar sight in my village. I've never thought about her looks particularly. She's a quiet, brown-haired girl with a pleasant manner who doesn't draw attention to herself. I had never thought of her as overweight, but she's been to a diet class and lost weight, probably only a stone as she wasn't fat in the first place. It's transformed her. She's become confident, glowing with health and vitality. Even her hair seems shinier.

What particularly struck me was her midriff. On so many of us this stretch between the bra and waist is lost in love handles. For her that's all gone. There's length and elegance there instead. Her clothes hang well. She looks easy in her skin.

I'd like a midriff.

MY MOTHER WAS not only a fantastic cook but also a constant, persistent, committed overeater. Even this is confusing to consider. She taught me to enjoy food. She loved to cook for us all and often made big celebratory meals for vast numbers of friends and family. She would wake early and launch into a great bout, calling instructions up the stairs, chopping, steaming and boiling, reducing, roasting and seasoning, until the table was laden with food.

In daily life she was often distracted but in this sphere she was completely focused and purposeful. Everyone was roped in. 'Darling, can you make me a huge vat of white sauce?' or 'I need these almonds slivered, but they must be paper thin, almost transparent, exactly like this.'

Some of my happiest times with her were when she was caught up in preparations for a party. It was in any case impossible to resist. If I refused to help, her blue eyes would register shock and her voice would wobble and falter, sadness and loss etched on her whole being. She would slump. Her reactions were always writ large. Although I often felt manipulated, her real need (neediness?) meant the manipulations worked. How could I turn my back? It would be too unkind.

As a young adult post-university, I used to visit her, determined not to repeat the patterns of childhood and overeat with her. Before getting home I would feel certain that I had changed and moved on, meaning to demonstrate the difference by maintaining my own choice of eating behaviour. After all, I was thinner than I had been in my teens, more in control.

As I stepped through the door she would appear like a whirlwind, draped in a cloud of purple, and apologise for not having a 'grand lunch' ready.

'Do you mind awfully if we just have soup and bread and cheese? I've made some fabulous borscht. I know it's a bit simple but there's lovely Camembert and a baguette, and some divine cream cakes too.'

Fine. Except this meant mounds of cheese, slabs of butter slathered onto fresh white bread, cream, butter, cheese, cream … You get the picture. Her favourite sandwich was in fact two slices of cheese with a chunk of butter between them. And all dressed up as a 'simple' lunch of soup and bread and cheese, what could be more innocent than that?

I would try hard to resist, this being far more calories than I wanted to consume. But minutes inside the door I would find myself heading to the kitchen to join the fat fest. Now I come to think of it, I can't imagine why. It was as if I was programmed to fit into her pattern and perhaps that's exactly what it was: a massive unconscious impulse that I literally couldn't resist.

Underneath her cheerful facade, my mother was determined that I join in and eat what she ate. If I didn't, it was a rejection and she was downcast, although the reasons were never explicit. If I did, she was exultant but I would leave with a headache, disappointed in myself, wondering when I would ever grow up.

A battle of wills, but of the most curious sort. It was as if she needed my participation to ratify her choices. And as if, in order to become myself, I needed to resist by defeating her in some unexplained way. Which was impossible to do because it would have hurt her so badly.

When it was time to go, she would come to the door with me, attention already wandering, follow me up the garden path to the gate, absent-mindedly deadheading flowers along the way and talking non-stop about neighbours I didn't know. No mention of the food behaviour that for me dominated the visit.

'You know – Becky and Shane! From the red house opposite the garage. They've got canaries. And two little boys, very sweet. They put an offer on that house in the square with the green shutters, you know the one, yes you do – think about it – but they were gazumped, and do you know who did it? Go on, guess ...' Never mind that they'd moved to the village after I left home and I'd never met them.

'Anyway, they've bought one of the cottages near the station, so now they're moving. It's such a shame. We'll miss them! Darling. So lovely to see you.' She would lean forward for a kiss, her fleshy cheek smelling of talcum powder and roses. She was cheered by my visit, I could tell. But I was furious with myself for giving in yet again.

NOW HERE I am, carefully examining how to approach weight loss, thinking of her with love and sorrow, and immediately hungry. There's a bit of rebellion in this – as soon as I get the first pangs of hunger, I resent the feeling and want to satisfy it straight away. There's also some panic. Perhaps the sky will fall in if I don't eat. And a bit of childishness – I work so hard/am so tired/am so dutiful, why shouldn't I? What I must learn to do is to count to ten before I do anything.

More than anything else, though, I've come to see that this automatic hunger reaction is programming. She programmed me to overeat with her. Nearly thirty years after her death that conditioning is still kicking in even at the memory of her. So this is my fight back (after all, it can't hurt her now). If you can be programmed to overeat, you can also reset the dial.

Here's an exercise which combines distress tolerance and mindfulness: I wait till I next feel hungry and decide to eat a banana. Only I don't eat it, I put it on the table in front of me. I wait, not one or two, but a full ten minutes and then eat it. Each day I stretch this gap by a few minutes. What I'm doing is not just mindful eating, I'm practising frictionless restraint: restraint without suffering. I'm concentrating on that small gap in time and learning to welcome it, not fear or resent it. My hope is that eventually it'll come naturally. I'm unpicking the pattern. Instead of reaching for a snack whenever I think of her, I'll smile and say, 'Wasn't she a great story teller?'

THE PERIOD OF waiting that lay between the arguments with Chris and gathering strength to act seemed to go on forever.

He had not completely given up his campaign against my obesity. He recognised that, like many serial dieters, my theory was good but my ability to put knowledge into practice was poor. His conclusion was that I should try therapy again. I had done it before to great effect, but every instinct told me that this time it wasn't the way to go. He insisted that my troubles were psychological. I argued hotly that they weren't. I conceded that I had conditioned myself over years to use food as a prop and that I needed to unlearn those habits, but I maintained that it was a cognitive problem rather than a psychological one – it just needed rethinking. I felt pressured and resentful and didn't believe it was his business to nag me.

I see now that my position was entirely defensive. When Chris brought up the subject, I was far from understanding how much I had been programmed by my mother. His prompts may well have been a painful echo of her manoeuvres, although in the opposite direction.

He started asking our friends if they didn't agree with him that I should lose weight. Maggie listened amazed and said to him, 'Oh don't be so silly,' which I took to be a vote in support of me. She wouldn't be drawn into further discussion.

Dan, a farmer friend of his said, 'You can't make up her mind for her – and anyway she's not that big,' which Chris hated because he felt my obesity was obvious for all to see. He thought Dan was sidestepping out of tact, and that his own position was rational: I was at risk of ill health and it was his job to talk me into changing. He couldn't understand why Maggie and Dan didn't back him up.

He told me about these conversations looking for sympathy, can you believe it, because they had gone nowhere. I was dumbfounded. I really couldn't believe his nerve. Weight is such a tender, taboo subject. The idea that he would canvass our friends for support on an issue so personal to me was astonishing. Not so much 'reader, I married him' as 'reader, I nearly divorced him!'

We seemed deadlocked. Out of desperation, we went to couples counselling – for two whole sessions. Our guy, Steve, had a bit of a paunch. When we described our problem to him, he patted his beer belly and said, 'Really? Well, I like a pasty.' Chris wanted to punch him.

Steve questioned us closely about what was wrong with our marriage. We agreed that we weren't struggling with the usual – money, sex, family or work.

'Just weight?' He seemed incredulous.

I suppose we were a bit confusing. We presented a pretty united front. We made each other laugh and agreed about how to describe the situation. He said that to him our marriage looked strong but that of course he must take our problem seriously.

'This is your situation as I see it. You can stay the same, change or separate.'

Chris was disgusted. He said later that if he'd wanted a bit of homespun philosophy he could have gone down the pub for it. It was tough on him and left him nowhere to go. He felt alone with his anxieties and misunderstood.

But for me it was different. Steve, like our friends, didn't think Chris had the right or responsibility to tell me what to do or try to supply motivation for me. I felt supported. I was still angry at the thin bint remark, and the threat, and the alcoholic analogy. But we kept talking and eventually I became less cross and began to listen to what he was saying. Later still, he stopped talking about it, finally realising that I had meant it when I had asked him not to.

In one of our last painful dog walks airing this subject I said to him, 'Wouldn't it be amazing if all that had to happen is for you to shut up about it, and for me to get on with it?'

He's quoted that back to me many times. At the time he didn't believe that I would make any changes. Truthfully, neither did I. But look – I have. I am.

EVERY SENTENCE AT the moment is apt to begin 'Kahneman says . . .' He's my new idol. His book isn't fast reading, that's for sure, but the implications of his research are profound.

For example, he writes about how energy-consuming it is to think with 'system 2'. He set a group of subjects a small task that was mentally challenging and noted that their energy level, and therefore ability to complete the task, was greatest at the beginning and fell away over time. He then gave some of them a sugary drink and others a diet drink. The performance of those who'd had sugar improved significantly whereas those who'd had sugar replacement did not.

This tells us that mental effort is hard work and that we can't keep it up for a sustained period without being fed. Ironic, if what we are trying to think about is rationing how much we eat. This could become a vicious circle – I think hard about overeating and how to avoid it, thinking hard makes me hungry, I eat to compensate for the lost energy, back to square one.

Kahneman says that both self-control and cognitive effort are mental work. The brain requires glucose to function and in a study where people were asked to remember a seven-digit sequence and afterwards offered a slice of chocolate cake or a bowl of fruit salad, they were more likely to choose the chocolate cake. 'The evidence suggests that you would be more likely to select the tempting chocolate cake when your mind is loaded with digits. System 1 has more influence on behaviour when system 2 is busy, and it has a sweet tooth.'

Also, if you have a series of mentally stressful decisions to make or mental work to do, the decision to resist a certain kind of food drops down the hierarchy. If that temptation becomes the last in a series of energy-consuming thought processes, then it's much more likely that you will give in to it. You simply don't have the mental energy to resist. Well there you are – all these years I've just been too busy thinking hard to resist temptation. Why is every dieter not told this?

I've known since I was twenty how I ought to eat, and yet I've been unable to do it. Is this why? When I told myself I work too hard/think too much/have too much else on – perhaps I was right? At the time it felt as if I just couldn't take on one more thing (a diet). Truthfully, I have always suspected that this line of thought was a form of denial but perhaps it was not. Perhaps it was based in some instinctive knowledge of my own mental processes, and what I really needed to do was to wind down some of those other activities to make space for healthy lifestyle choices.

In my mid-fifties, I'm a ripe old age to be working all this stuff out. I don't believe that's because I'm especially dim or lazy. In fact the statistics bear out (not just for me, but for everyone) that it's exceptionally hard to lose weight, even harder to keep it off. It really has been a long and tortuous road and I really have tried. I suspect the answer is that I just haven't been thinking about it the right way. Looking ahead, the question is, how can I protect myself from mental energy dips so as not to carry on with the same poor eating decisions? Food for thought indeed.

To fight this particular demon has always seemed to me to require extreme self-control and a kind of mental toughness which I just didn't appear to have. Maybe that was all wrong. Perhaps it's about getting enough sleep, reducing other stresses and learning patience. Wouldn't it be crazy if it was that simple?

On the day that I started all this and weighed in at seventeen stone plus, I didn't know what my new approach should be. The failures of the past loomed over me and I was anxious not to repeat them. Desperate to succeed this time, I made a kind of inventory of what I could bring to the table. High on the list was my background as a researcher and I decided to use that skill to the max on this, one of the most difficult and privately stressful areas of my life.

For the first time in a long time I was also fully committed. I had often mouthed the words that expressed a desire to lose weight, but flaked out as soon as it got tough. This time I've set a realistic timeframe and settled in for the long haul.

Recognising that weight is a very emotive subject, I decided to do everything I could to reduce that emotionality. I wanted to learn some objectivity, treat it like a project, and get better at it.

I am still committed to that approach. Every time I get stuck, I look it up and find a new strategy. Every time I slip, I forgive myself and move on. And every time it gets really hard, I visit Bridget.

Sobering fact #9: *Parent weight change is related to child weight change. Family-based behavioural treatments are among the most successful for paediatric obesity while parental obesity may increase the risk of a child becoming obese.*

JAMA Paediatrics, 2004

CHAPTER 10

Reversal of fortune

15st 7lb

Saturday, 1 October 2011

It's easier to climb to the top of the tor than when I started. I'm two stone lighter, so it ought to be. When I get there, an astonishing sight hits me right between the eyes.

Bridget's skipping. And she's surprisingly nimble.

'Hello, what's this?' I think she might stop, embarrassed, but she's too busy counting steps, and giggling.

'Exercise? I didn't think you did exercise?'

She's breathless but full of gusto and carries right on, her wild hair spinning out round her head.

She's having fun. No point in stopping her with my worries, so I give her a cheery wave and retrace my steps. There's always next time.

This scene leaves me with a question – if she exercises, why don't I?

Answers come thick and fast: because I don't want to. Because I don't like it. Because I bustle about, busy and active. Because, if I eat moderately enough, I won't have to.

It's a shame that Bridget is so occupied. She might have something to say about these instant reactions to the very thought of exercise.

I'M NOT AWARE of having gone off plan this week but even so I've put on a pound. This is the first time I've gained in four months. In times past, this small gain would have counted as a disaster, possibly even a reason to give up. There's a distant voice of rebellion in me now. I've stuck to my diet, and it hasn't worked! How can this be? It's just not fair. I note this reaction but do not give way to it.

Mentally, I've really struggled over the last few days and I don't know why. Could it be because more people have started to notice I've lost weight? I want to send my unconscious a message to say, 'Hang on in there, don't worry, nothing bad will come of this, it's going to be OK.'

A long slow diet is always praised by health professionals as the best and only desirable way to achieve permanent weight loss. That's easy to say but much harder to do. Every now and then it occurs to me to try a quicker method. I could be done with it, fixed once and for all. £5000–£15,000 for a stomach staple, gastric bypass or gastric band, and as long as the surgery didn't go wrong, job done. Why not?

Quite apart from the health risks and the cost, the answer is obvious to me. It's because it wouldn't fix my mind. The desire to eat is in my head, not my stomach. I would still want to eat the way I did before. There are plenty of stories of people who have had surgery and still manage to consume enough to keep them obese. I could well be one of them, but even if I wasn't my thinking wouldn't change just because I had had a gastric band. I would be hungry in my head but full in my stomach. That sounds grim.

Face it, all surgery does is to remove some of the pleasures of eating. I would still have to rethink the way I eat. Gastric constriction just takes away some of the opportunities for binging, which is not even one of my problems, so I've talked myself out of it. I'm cutting out the risky and expensive surgical procedure and teaching myself to reconsider my attitude to food instead.

In 2010 I produced a film about Albert Goering, the anti-Nazi brother of Hermann Goering. He helped scores of Jews and others escape from Nazi Germany. His moving story is one of huge bravery which, far from being rewarded, landed him in prison for several years after the war for the dubious crime of 'being Hermann Goering's brother'. He was eventually released, based on the testimonies of some of the people he had helped to escape from Germany during the war.

He has one surviving child, a daughter, who lives in South America. She flew to Germany to film with us. She has had a gastric band but it hasn't helped her to lose weight. She explained that to get around it, and continue to consume to her heart's content, she went for liquid foods, with the result that she was still obese.

She is a lovely, empathetic, generous woman. Late one night we sat in a bar together next to our hotel. A few toddies to see us to sleep? No. She was drinking zabaglione, an Italian dessert, like warm alcoholic custard, through a straw. She took both my hands in hers and looked me over, weighing me up, comparing my size to hers (I was heavy then, but I'm guessing she had four or five stone on me) and looked intently at me.

'Don't be like me. Just do it, just lose the weight naturally. You can, you know. Just do it.' I took this as kindness itself. I think of her often.

I decide to imagine that I've had the operation, and eat accordingly. I've said it before – this is cheaper and safer than surgery.

ABOUT A YEAR before I met Chris I got down to 10st 8lb, the lightest I have been as an adult. At that point in my career I was a freelance television researcher. I landed a dream job travelling halfway round the world filming a series about the Victorian plant hunters. The crew set off to shoot the first half of the trip while I researched the second half. Six weeks later I met up with them on the other side of the world. I was already good friends with the producer and his PA, who I had worked with for months leading up to the shoot, but the rest of the crew were new to me.

All tanned to walnut brown from a stint in Polynesia en route, they were very welcoming and made me feel part of the team right away. Paul, the cameraman, and the sound recordist Duncan were especially kind. Being young and naive, I didn't quite get the tone of this friendliness immediately.

If anything, I preferred Duncan. Despite what I took to be a bit of normal shoot flirting, I suppose I felt safer with him because I knew he was married. I told you I was naive.

Weeks later, I was by chance alone with Paul, bumping round the back streets of Mumbai in a cronky old bus when suddenly, from absolutely nowhere as it seemed to me, he said, 'OK darlin', you going to give me a bonk or what?'

I was completely taken aback. 'Thanks for the offer, very kind of you, but no, actually.' Why I felt the need to be polite I don't know.

'You gonna give Dunc one?'

I shook my head.

He sniffed. 'I guess that's quits then.'

I raised my eyebrows, not following.

'Dunc an' me had a bet before you got here. To see who could get you into bed first. Obviously we hadn't seen you then. If you was fat it was gonna be off.'

Of course it was gonna be off. Why wouldn't it be? This wasn't about actual attraction, or my fabulous personality. It was a bet. Because they'd both lost, I had to be humiliated a little by having the bet revealed to me. If I had slept with one of them, presumably they'd have done their best to keep it secret from me.

It didn't even occur to me to answer in kind. But what immediately went through my mind was a crisp but silent summing up. 'You're rough, dumb and sexist and your only redeeming quality is that you can be funny sometimes. Hell would freeze over before I'd ever sleep with you.'

He had propositioned me only because I was thin. He wouldn't have looked twice at me a couple of stone heavier, where I was more used to being. But far from feeling flattered, I was outraged. I like to think that a young woman these days would not have held back from saying so.

Sexism. There's so much to say about it, and it all seems so obvious that I can hardly bring myself to address it. When that sort of coercive and degrading behaviour is commonplace, it's no wonder that some of us see being thin as a mixed blessing and our bodies resort to a defensive position. If being fat meant no longer being the object of that kind of attention, it seemed my body had taken matters into its own hands and said, 'Bring it on.'

In those days I lived in Bristol. When the trip was over, I went to see Julie, a dancer and masseuse. I showed off my new body, confident that she'd be interested and impressed, and she didn't fail me. I undressed, she pushed and pulled, admired and tweaked.

'It's great. You must be really pleased with yourself,' she said. 'Now, I guess you just need to lose a little more off your bottom. Is that what you're thinking?'

From where I am now, I realise how much I must have achieved to hear that from her. She belonged to the cult of the body perfect. If she thought I just had a bit to trim off my bottom, from her that was praise indeed. Probably I'd done superbly well. But my heart plummeted at her words. 'It's never going to be enough,' I thought. 'It doesn't matter how hard I try, the goal is always going to be out of reach.'

There is a piece of wisdom that goes 'what makes us is what we make of what others make of us'. There was nothing wrong in what she said, but there was a big problem in my reaction to it. I took it badly, as a sign of failure, and despaired just when I should have been celebrating. How much I had also been bruised by the crew bet, I can't really tell.

This sinking of the heart crystallised when I stood in front of my bathroom mirror and gazed at 10st 8lb. A thought bubbled up from nowhere, rising to my mind like verbal tumbleweed at the sight of my trimmed-down body.

'You don't deserve to look like that,' I said to myself.

It was not immediately obvious to me how pernicious and self-destructive this thought was. Very soon after this I met Chris and when I told him about this experience, he fiercely denied that I didn't 'deserve' to be thin and seemed almost angry that I should think that way. But slowly I began to put weight on again. I have never got anywhere near that same healthy weight for my height since.

Chris has often referred back to that incident. He thought it was a key moment. Gradually, as I got heavier, he began to understand how deep-rooted my weight problem was and after a year or two he came to the conclusion that I would benefit from seeing a therapist to 'deal with it'. He thought that when I was resolved about other issues, my weight would naturally drop and right itself. Initially reluctant, out of fear I think, eventually I agreed. Despite my anxieties, it turned out to be a fantastically constructive process, helping me to resolve many of my childhood issues. Through this work I began to feel more whole, less conflicted and closer to being at peace. But nothing had changed with my weight.

When is it ever going to change? Every dieter knows the despair of thinking that. When is it going to change? The answer is right here, right now, on this page.

Sobering fact #10: *In 2000, about 37,000 bariatric surgeries were performed in the United States. By 2013, the number had risen to 220,000.*

Harriet Brown, *Body of Truth*, 2015

CHAPTER 11

Doing the maths

15st 0lb

Saturday, 22 October 2011

How is Bridget? Trucking on, contemplative, not to be disturbed.

I sit beside her fire and talk to her while she busies herself around the place.

'I've had two lots of friends to stay recently,' I tell her. 'I cooked for them, drank a bit with them, had a great time – and then tightened my belt after they'd gone. I'm learning.'

She barely listens, padding back and forth with her wheelbarrow, nodding occasionally. But she seems content.

THIS WEEK I'VE been on austerity measures, which means meagre portions, no extras. The result is that I've lost four pounds in one week, bringing the total to just over two stone so far. Four pounds is a big loss in so short a time, especially several months into a diet, perhaps too much. I'll go easier next week.

'Never satisfied,' says Maggie. 'Usually it's not enough – this time you say it's too much in one go. Be happy.'

I am happy, but mindful that four pounds a week is not sustainable.

That means I'm making progress, but I've been here so many times before that there's no room for complacency. It's a tentative start, that's all I'll allow. And I'm on the cusp of another milestone. The last time I was under fifteen stone was before I was pregnant with Orlando. It feels like I'm turning back the clock.

Sunday, 23 October 2011

AS SO OFTEN after a good result, the next day I have a really hard day. It's a Sunday and there isn't work to keep me busy and distract me. All day I struggle and battle with myself, wanting to visit the kitchen cupboard and graze. Placate myself with a few crackers with ultra-thin slivers of cheese, or a Ryvita with a scraping of jam and thin slivers of banana, a good controllable snack. It never feels quite filling enough – but then, what would be? In that mood, nothing.

I hold on to that thought. My mind is whispering to me to eat – go on, just a slice of bread and jam, just a couple of biscuits, just, just, just ... But I know the truth: this particular sort of hunger is never satisfied. Whatever I eat, I will still want to eat more. It is perpetual fire. The best technique to quench it is to do nothing. Eat nothing. Sit on my hands. Keep still. Stay with the feelings, but do not act on them. So, as I say, a struggle, but I limp through and survive with not much damage done.

At the moment my Google homepage and Facebook timeline are both littered with pop-up adverts promising me dramatic weight loss. 'Lose 3 stone in a month!' 'Diet tips doctors won't tell you!' 'The diet that only celebs know!' I've checked, and the young researchers at work don't get bombarded with this nonsense. How did they find me – surely the weight loss sites I subscribe to haven't sold my contact details to random advertisers? Or do search engines and social media simply assume that a woman of my age must be concerned about being fat?

For me, they're a private source of fun. I look at them, know they promise the earth and deliver nothing, and secretly think, 'On it. Doing it. Already there mate.'

I'm being disciplined, and sticking to a weekly weigh-in, because jumping on the scales too often seems like a bad idea. Bodies seem to be vague fluid shapes whose weight fluctuates all over the place, like balloons full of water being tethered in a swimming pool, bobbing and weaving about. At any given point we get a rough approximation of our body weight. We must take into consideration not just the time of day and what we're wearing but how much we've drunk, whether we've just eaten and the state of bladder and bowels. So any one day's result is really a sort of average weight, not definitive, and not to be completely relied upon. If you have a tidy mind none of this is very satisfactory, but it's all we have.

Chris says it reminds him of the speedometer in the family car when he was a kid. In those days the needle did not move smoothly round the dial as they do now, but wobbled back and forth around a speed that could be anywhere from 23mph to 35mph. You had to guess by taking a rough average.

In the case of the scales, that wobbling motion can last over days. Or the opposite: Chris weighed himself the other day, drank a glass of water, then weighed again. He was two pounds heavier. 'That's not possible,' he barked, 'that water didn't weigh two pounds.' He was indignant. 'That flies in the face of physics!' Every dieter will surely have had similar experiences.

I'd prefer an A + B = C kind of body where I could predict exactly what would happen if I ate this, and avoided that, but it doesn't work that way. The body has a rhythm of its own which is quite different from how we think it should behave. We imagine that we should be able to regulate what happens to our weight precisely, but of course we can't.

Despite hundreds of thousands of studies on obesity, it is still far from fully understood. Not the causes, not the solutions. We have some clues, that's the best we can say.

If only there was a monitor which could assess us from head to toe, consumption, exercise, every aspect of our physical condition, and could tell us definitively what to eat and drink in order to lose weight. I imagine a combined pedometer, food and drink monitor and metabolism checker. Whoever invents that gadget will make a billion. Till it comes, I'm on my own slow path to recovery.

There are of course various fitness trackers on the market but they can't yet accurately track calories in and calories out. A recent two-year study in the USA presented alarming findings for the makers of such equipment. Two hundred and sixteen overweight adults were put on a low calorie diet. After six months, half of them were given a fitness monitoring system to chart their progress, including an armband to track exercise, backed up by an app to log their consumption. The other half of the group were asked to monitor their own diet and exercise without technology to help.

Both groups lost weight, but the technology-free set lost nearly twice as much (13lb versus 7.7lb) as those who scrutinised every step electronically. The suspicion was that the monitors provided a false sense of security to dieters who were actually more effective at doing the job by themselves.

But if the monitors did a more comprehensive job, that might not be the case.

THIS HAS BEEN a week of upset and upheaval. I am sitting in a room with someone I am very fond of who is furious with me, and taking it like a woman. One of our regular producers, Jeannie, is at the end of her contract. She's stressed by events at home and wants a break, but she doesn't want us to hire anyone else to work on our next series. She says she will feel replaced. This is not rational but she's a dear colleague and I hate to see her sad and angry. But I can't give in to this. We are busier than ever, and we need someone to do her work while she's away.

Why mention it? Because I'm dwelling on those irritating magazine articles again: *identify the emotional triggers that cause you to overeat* ... This is definitely an emotionally charged situation. The more she says the more reasons I find to be indignant, defensive and angry, and try to resist them all. I keep remembering the pressures of her situation, caring for a mother with Alzheimer's who no longer recognises her. I try to offer support and clarity in equal measure and not to react angrily whatever the provocation. This is easier said than done, but it's important.

I feel blamed, and over the next few days it becomes obvious that I am indeed being held responsible – for what? Acting reasonably and I believe in the best interests of all, but still it's horrible to see someone I am close to hurt and to know that she's angry with me.

I am sad and sorry, but it isn't a reason to stuff my face. I watch like a hawk to see what happens, but it doesn't seem to be having a bad effect. That might be because I'm looking out for stress eating (a better phrase than 'comfort eating' because there's nothing comforting about overeating) and vigilance is heading off the impulse.

A FLASHBACK TO my mother teaching me to make fudge. I'm six, and we are living in a village in Somerset. Her latest boyfriend has not come home the night before. He was playing away in the most public manner possible with a girl he'd met in the village pub.

I have a sugar thermometer in my hand, measuring the exact temperature of the melting heap of soft brown sugar, now just liquid. Too hot and it'll turn to caramel, then toffee. I bend over the saucepan, concentrating hard on all that boiling sweetness.

My mother is a good teacher. She lets me handle the thermometer and the sugar with only a little nerviness. Her eyes fill as she explains the difference between the stages, soft ball, hard ball, crack. Every now and then she gives me a sudden fierce hug. She brushes her hand across the eyes and tells me to butter the dish to set the fudge in. Finally, her tears spill over and she sobs. She says, 'Darling, tell me he'll come back to me.'

I'm torn. I've been put in this situation too often before. Murmuring support, I add milk and butter, and keep stirring. There's a certain clinical edge in the way I deal with her. I don't want her to suffer, but I don't want to hear about it. And I really want to learn how to make fudge.

CHRIS IS CAUTIOUSLY encouraging at the moment. He asks how I'm managing and I tell him about Bridget. I explain that I'm trying to tackle my own hidden motivations for overeating by visualising her and speaking to her directly. He's intrigued, so I go on.

I ask him if he has ever had the experience of eating before thinking and his first reaction is 'no'. But on reflection he describes taking three chocolate biscuits from the cupboard to have with a cup of tea, making the cup of tea and then looking for the biscuits. Literally scouring the kitchen – 'Must have put them down, where are they?' Only to find the wrappers screwed up in the bin. 'There you are,' I say, 'that's the Cadover Bridge Syndrome.'

For Chris this scenario is nothing like as charged as it is for me because he doesn't have a weight problem. Hence the original 'no' when I asked the question. If you're just wondering where you put your biscuits down, with no additional baggage, it's not a big deal to find evidence of your own unconscious eating. If you're grappling with a long-term weight problem, it is.

'My advice to you,' I told him – and don't think I didn't enjoy this – 'is to stretch the time between deciding to have the biscuit and actually eating it. Make the tea first. Get the biscuits out and carry them to the table. Get your cup, carry the teapot to the table. The biscuits are still there. Sit down and eat them, savouring them. Be mindful. That way you'll enjoy them more and you'll remember you've done it too.'

The terrible cheat about the Cadover Bridge Syndrome is that when you eat in a dreamlike state, spurred on by your unconscious, you don't even taste what you're putting in your mouth, let alone enjoy it. By the time you're even aware that you've done it, the food is long gone. If it's pleasure in food you're after, that sort of sleep-eating is a dead loss on every count.

Discussing my weight with Chris has become easier than at any time in our marriage – easier for me, anyway. For him it's a bit more complicated. With the wind in my sails I've suddenly become very vocal on the subject and gabble away, eager to share my strategies and challenges.

He reminds me of a cat that's miffed because you've been on holiday – delighted when you come back, but then turns its back to punish you, taking its time before it forgives you. I had told Chris he wasn't welcome to raise my weight issue with me because hearing his opinion about it was demoralising and painful. He stopped but felt silenced. Now that's all changed and I'm keen to talk, there's a part of him that wants to say, 'No, you told me not to speak to you about your weight, so I won't. And I'm not listening to you burble on either.'

Luckily another part of him is more generous-spirited and indulges me, even if with a slightly sardonic edge. But I get that.

Sobering fact #11: *Overweight and obese children are significantly more likely to be obese in adulthood.*

World Health Organization, 2017

CHAPTER 12

Visualisation

14st 13lb

Saturday, 12 November 2011

'Bridget, where are you?' It's dark and cold, a howling wind whipping round the tor, and I can't find her, although I know she's there somewhere.

'Come out, come out, wherever you are.' I should know by now that it doesn't work to badger or complain, to hector or lecture her into being.

The only way to contact her is to defocus, breathe deep and think. Where is she? What is she? She's a spirit, an idea, a gift, a messenger, an avatar, an icon, an ideal, a beacon, a companion, a fellow traveller, a friend.

But she's not my servant, and she's not at my beck and call. She doesn't have to come if she doesn't want to. I can't make her.

I'm a little lost and could do with some help.

I leave a note for her on the wood pile. 'Came. Couldn't find you. Missed you.' It feels like connection of a sort.

STILL ON PLAN, have cut back on fruit to keep calories in check, but it's very slow. I feel thinner but am stuck as a stuck thing. Be-plateaued. One pound off in a month, none for three weeks. And that one pound off, three weeks ago, was hard wrung. It felt like a great achievement, not so much in a physical sense, but as a victory over the emotions. The thought of surrender and failure flickers through from time to time, only to be dismissed. I'm grateful that I still feel whole-hearted. It would be so easy to give in.

Bethan is a freelance graphic designer who often works with us. She's struggled with her weight in the past but not in the same way as me. Her issue is that she can lose too much and she hints of borderline anorexia in the past. Now she is in a happy relationship and settled at work she has pulled back from it and her partner Dan is kind and vigilant. He makes sure she eats. These days, too, she recognises the early warning signs and takes care not to go there. Although our issues are opposites in a way, mirror images of each other, we bond over them. She takes a close interest in my efforts and, when I complain of being becalmed, she offers an idea – that a diet can become too predictable, which in turn can slow the metabolism. The daily rhythm of my meals has become very regular so this seems plausible to me.

'Give it a kick up the jacksie!' she says. 'Go right off piste, not mental, but surprise yourself.'

There's a stray thought that she might be throwing me off, sending me up a blind alley for reasons more connected with her own eating disorder than my welfare. But sensing her warmth and positivity, I banish this negative idea and decide that she might have a point. So I eat a Milky Way, followed by chips in the evening. Before you think I've lost the plot, all this is in counted, tiny portions, contained and accounted for within my diet. It remains to be seen whether it'll actually do any good though.

THIS PLATEAU FEELS like a physical problem. But is there really such a thing? I've always thought it must be a purely psychological phenomenon, a myth in scientific terms. But recent research into leptin levels suggests that the plateau might have some basis in reality after all.

Leptin is a hormone which was first discovered in the mid-1990s. Its primary function is to regulate the body's response to food intake and to maintain energy balance. When the body's fat stores are replenished, it sends a 'fullness' message to the brain to dial down hunger, which in turn stops us eating. This is one way that it works to maintain body weight.

However, when food is scarce (starvation or dieting) it has another role. It can alter the metabolism to make maximum use of the scant fat stores available. In other words, it slows the metabolism down, again for the sake of maintaining body weight. Allegedly five to six months into a diet is where this kick to the metabolism usually hits – almost bang on where I am now.

For us dieters, this is very bad news. We don't want to maintain body weight, we want to change it. But it looks as though our own bodies may be working against our efforts. There is a ring of truth about this theory because it matches not just my own experience but anecdotes from many other dieters too.

However, leptin's functions are not yet fully understood. In the field of science a discovery from the 1990s is considered relatively new and further research is still underway. Most articles conclude frustratingly by saying that we will have to wait and see how leptin works and what else it does.

That means there isn't much useful advice available about breaking through a plateau. So, this week's technique is to follow Bethan's advice and shock the system with new foods. I'm sceptical, but interested to see whether it works.

Meanwhile Bridget and I seem to be doing well. I've been back to see her and found her quite easily. When I asked where she had disappeared to, she was non-committal, but friendly. We're back on track.

I'M TRYING TO visualise myself into a new size and shape to help me think myself into the right frame of mind. My wardrobe is stuffed full of clothes from every era of my life, sizes

12–22 inclusive. I rarely chuck any away. You never know when you might grow back into them. Unfortunately.

The reason that I'm scrabbling through the back of the wardrobe like this is that a study out this week shows that we are all more suggestible than previously thought. Apparently we are very porous and open to influence, particularly from visual cues. If there's a mobile phone on a table in front of us, chances are that we won't bond with the person we are sitting with. Even if the mobile is sitting on the table next to us it has a similar effect. Inspired by this research I'm trying out autosuggestion of a positive kind, using strong visual cues.

So I rummage through and try on lots of passionately loved old relics, starting with a dress I had when I was thirteen, pure 1960s hype: it's a perfect flower power mini dress in great swirls of colour, pink, orange and yellow, very *Ab Fab*, such a classic that it should really have ended up in a costume collection. Still too small and so very short it's hard to believe I ever wore it outside the house – but I did.

There's a pair of dark green jodhpurs that I lived in for a year or so in the mid-1980s. They're in great condition. I thought they were part of a fat phase but they're tiny! They come up to my thighs, but no further.

Which are the clothes I'd still like to wear? A pair of black Levi's, button fly, which I haven't worn for nearly twenty years. I remember I bought them around the time I went to see Julie, the dancer-cum-masseur, she of the body perfect. Because I had just lost a lot of weight, I didn't know what size I was. I tucked myself into the tiny changing room of a cool and intimidating boutique and tried on one pair after another. The Cinderella moment came with this pair. I can still feel the shock of being able to get into a thirty-two-inch waist. I came out of that dressing room walking on air.

Then there's a pair of stretch leggings covered in red roses that I wore the day after I got married. Size 16 but very forgiving – they won't take long to get back into.

At the back of the wardrobe is a 1950s prom dress I used to wear to parties – black taffeta daubed with big pale pink roses. Also a pale grey suit with silk lining that was made for me at my lightest in about 1986. The material is Next furnishing fabric, grey brocade, with charcoal grey velvet lapels. The skirt is very short, the height of fashion when it was made. Some good fairy whispered in my ear and made me ask for a huge hem – probably four inches – so come the day that I can get into it, I can let it down and wear it. I will wear it.

Last and greatest favourite of all, there's a pair of size 12 printed velvet Benetton trousers, circa 1989. At the time they were worn with a fine white lawn blouse with a lace collar and high heels. It's hard to believe I will ever wear those again, but a distant voice murmurs – you could, you might, maybe …

Turns out I'm already back into the red rose-covered leggings.

Orlando is incredulous. 'What do you think you look like?' he splutters. 'They're ludicrous!' Yes, I think, he's probably right. 'But they're so mad, you sort of get away with it.' He's a lovely boy.

Next I try the Levi's. Two stone ago I couldn't get them past my knees. Now they come all the way up but they won't do up.

The prom dress cheers me. It gapes by only about three inches. I can imagine it back on. I think hard. I remember wearing it to an exhibition opening at an art gallery in Bristol. I was slightly in love with someone there who had been involved with a friend of mine. I knew it was over for her. She dumped him at this party and I hugged him.

'Don't,' he said, and that one word carried more meaning than any one word should be able to. It was forbidding. But the next day he called and asked me out. I was heady with excitement and enjoyed the anticipation for a week.

For six months or so we had dates and walks, flirtation but no progression. It was doomed from the outset. Neither of us was ready to take the plunge and actually get involved.

The whole relationship could really be summed up in that first exchange, 'Don't.'

But I don't blame the dress. It is still a lovely thing. Vintage from the fifties, had another moment of glory in the eighties, now ripe for renovation.

The Benetton trousers of lost beauty I do not approach. I am not worthy.

The positive way forward is to visualise myself in these old favourites, not dwell on failure. No more swathes and layers of floating material. Clothes that fit and flatter – that's what I'm after now.

AN IMAGE OF whirling, swirling colours and textures, tent dresses like vast baby clothes – now who does that conjure up? I think back to her, a vision of extravagance, bright red henna-dyed hair, a reversible poncho (yes, they had a moment in the 1960s), fuchsia pink on one side and fiery orange on the other, marching up the street to my school gate. Standing next to me, watching, was a particularly rigid teacher who I really didn't like.

'Who is that extraordinary woman?' in tones of outrage.

'What on earth does she want?' practically spitting with indignation.

Bland response from me: 'That's my mother.'

Don't think I didn't enjoy that moment.

Miss O'Hara flushed a dark, brick red. She could never quite look me in the eye after that. Good.

14st 13lb

Saturday, 19 November 2011

AN ITEM ON the *Today* programme about obesity. If you lose just 10 per cent of your body weight, you dramatically decrease the likelihood of getting cancer, heart disease, stroke and diabetes. Done that.

The strange conclusion seemed to be that you should lose 10 per cent even if you can't do any more. But of course after the first 10 per cent, I just see another 10 per cent in front of me, ready to be shed.

Did the kick up the jacksie to my diet work? In a word, no. It was fun, a brief respite from unrelenting steamed vegetables, but no, it didn't jump-start my metabolism in the desired way. To be fair, I didn't put on any weight either, but in the absence of a positive shift, common sense told me to stop it after a day or so.

Am not dwelling on stuckness. There's no point. I've already decided not to waver or give in. As already admitted, I do know that the most sensible thing would be to start doing some exercise to shake things up, but fitting it into my lifestyle is tricky. I'm very busy and it's just too time-consuming. I think you could say there's some resistance here. Instead I stay steadfast to the programme, trusting that in the end I can do this by diet alone.

Before I began, it had never occurred to me that a person could go on a diet, keep it faithfully and still not lose weight. If someone else had told me they had done that, I would doubt them. I would question whether they were a) telling the truth or b) competent to count their calories. But now I've kept at it diligently for so long without success and I know from personal experience it's a real phenomenon.

But in the end the body must give in and lose weight.

My new mantra: 'It can't NOT work, in the end it MUST work.'

14st 13lb

Saturday, 26 November 2011

I'd like to say to Bridget, 'It's not a threat, there's no starvation round the corner, nothing worth hanging on to, come on Bridget, let it go …' but I'm not convinced you can talk your unconscious into collaborating. Mine seems to be particularly obdurate.

I FEEL AS though I've been shifting only ounces every week, but have just looked back and since the beginning of October I've lost eight pounds. So every time I write that nothing is shifting, nothing changing, I'm stuck and don't know what to do to keep it moving, PLEASE TAKE IT WITH A PINCH OF SALT.

It's obviously not true although, as you see, it is the running commentary in my brain.

The trick, as I've said, is to look only at two perspectives:

1. One day at a time.
2. Long-term.

The bit to avoid is the mid-term – where will I be in three weeks? Seven weeks? Because unfortunately our bodies are not chemistry sets and we can't predict exactly how much we'll lose in that period. Intermediate goals are therefore doomed to disappointment. Also, it's not good to encourage our own short-termism. This needs to be a permanent shift in how we think and live.

Now, sermon over. Yesterday I took a two-hour walk with Chris, Orlando and the dog. We got back in the dark and I was shattered, but perhaps it helped. Despite research findings that suggest it doesn't necessarily aid weight loss, I am reluctantly sure that exercise is the way to go. But I'm still resisting beastly spinning and blasted swimming. Must I? So so dull.

Sobering fact #12: *Research in both the UK and the US is emerging to show that exercise has a negligible impact on weight loss.*

Observer, 2010
Mintel, 2014

CHAPTER 13

Sibling rules

14st 10lb

Saturday, 3 December 2011

I wondered what Bridget would do about Christmas.

She has hung a wreath with a red ribbon threaded through it above her cave, and there are a few lighted red candles dotted round at the back. Still, I don't think Christmas is a big deal for her.

'I've got a present for you,' I say, handing her a perfect pine cone decorated like a miniature Christmas tree. She smiles and nods.

Her present for me? She touches my cheek with one finger. The gesture is clear – 'Wait and see!' it seems to say.

IN OUR LOFT we keep a huge cardboard box full of ancient, slightly moth-eaten but much-loved Christmas decorations. Each one has a story which I tell Orlando every year like a piece of oral history.

Hanging three elegant pointed drops, their colours almost rubbed off, 'These were brought down from London one Christmas by Mum's friend Ba. Once they were fluorescent pink, acid yellow and lime. They were so cool! We'd never seen anything like them. Now they're ghostly pale, faded from all the Christmases they've seen.'

A glass heart, plump and transparent. 'This one comes from my sister Belinda who died before you were born. She always gave me heart-shaped presents because my birthday is close to Valentine's Day – but I don't know where she found a heart-shaped Christmas tree bauble.'

A little wooden rocking horse, scarlet and gold. 'This was given to me by Diana, who had just had a baby on her own and gave a present to everyone she knew who helped her.'

A tatty angel with a wonky halo. 'My mum made this. She embroidered the dress with pearls, look, most of them have dropped off, but here's a few.' Passing sadness that he never met her. He feels it too.

And so on.

All the decorations have to go up on the tree every year. If I try to pass over one, Orlando objects. He says they'll feel left out.

THREE POUNDS OFF, all in one go. I'm as happy as a clam. It feels like a reward for good behaviour, but is obviously no such thing, just the result of relentless hard work done in small steps over a long period of time.

It's amazing how opinionated people are. They ask how it's going and I say, 'OK, but I was on a plateau for five weeks where I battled to keep the faith, and now I've lost three pounds in one week, no rhyme or reason.'

'Oh,' they say, knowledgably, 'you must have done more exercise this week.'

'No.'

'Or,' they say, 'unconsciously, you must have eaten less.'

'No, I track what I eat.'

'I expect you do,' they say, with a small smile – they know best. Maddening.

I wish all these experts who have never even attempted a long-term diet, let alone succeeded on one, would stop looking smug and knowing best. From a purely technical point of view, this is actually quite difficult, never mind the emotional, social and psychological issues that get in the way too.

Here's the law of diminishing returns as it applies to dieting: as you lose weight, you need fewer calories to maintain your body, therefore, to lose even more weight, you must keep reducing your calories. Some diets, like the one I'm on, deliberately start you on a generous allowance so that when the loss slows down, you have somewhere to go and can reduce your intake again without too much pain.

That's where I am now. Still losing, but much more slowly than at the beginning. Still moving on.

CURIOUS TO KNOW more about leptin, I dig deeper. One of the most remarkable things about the human body is its ability to regulate its own weight. At least some of the biological mechanisms responsible for this extraordinary feat are located within the tiny but powerful hypothalamus, an almond-sized area of the brain. One aspect takes the form of appetite regulation by two hormones: ghrelin, which controls hunger, and our friend leptin, which controls how full we feel. But leptin also has an influence on many other hormones which affect our weight including thyroid hormones, which regulate metabolism, cortisol (the 'stress hormone') and insulin, which regulates blood sugar.

So it appears that leptin is more than just a 'fullness hormone'. The clue is in the name: the word leptin comes from Greek, *leptos*, meaning thin, and it seems to have a wide-ranging responsibility for keeping weight down.

Oddly, though, obese people sometimes have raised levels of leptin but remain overweight. This has led to a theory that they may be suffering from leptin resistance, meaning that they stop getting the messages to tell them when they are full. Hence the desire to go on eating after everyone else has put down their fork.

One study tested the effect of injecting leptin into twenty-seven women whose weight had plateaued after bariatric surgery. After their surgeries, they had all lost weight initially but then stalled. The purpose of the study was to find out if giving them leptin could inhibit their hunger and allow them to lose more weight, but sixteen weeks of regular leptin injections had no discernible effect. Both the obese group and a control group, who had been given a placebo, lost at the same rate.

Slightly depressingly, this study was carried out to test whether leptin could be synthesised and used as a 'cure' for obesity. Obviously there is a huge commercial incentive to medicalise solutions to obesity. But the risk is that less invasive methods of treatment that do not offer the same profit motive may not be as well explored.

As well as those commercial pressures, there is a journalistic delight in reporting new studies with as much flourish as possible. I like a study as much as the next woman, but I try to treat the reportage of their findings with caution.

For example, I've seen articles declaring authoritatively that yo-yo dieting disrupts leptin levels, causing dieters to gain more weight than they lost in the first place. I haven't seen convincing evidence that this is so. It is true that the majority of dieters regain the weight they lost, and sometimes more. There the conclusive evidence peters out. Many reasons, apart from reduced levels of leptin, are suggested for the weight regain: slower metabolism post weight loss, expanded fat cells, lifestyle issues and genetic factors are all candidates. Throw psychology into the mix, and it's easy to see why weight loss is difficult to maintain.

But to declare yo-yo dieting as the 'cause' seems like fat-shaming of a rather sophisticated sort, since the implication is that dieting causes harm rather than aids health. The message is: you've damaged your health by becoming overweight and now you'll damage it further by trying to control that weight. Common sense tells us that is not so, because the statistics speak for themselves. There is undoubtedly a correlation between diabetes, stroke, heart disease (and more) and obesity, and reducing obesity lowers those risks, so the attempt to get to grips with it is surely unarguable.

14st 8lb

Friday, 23 December 2011

THIS WEEK IS my eldest brother Luke's seventieth birthday party. I wear a little black dress and some make-up (a rarity) and wonder if anyone will notice I'm two and a half stone lighter. There are photo montages of family and friends all around the room, including some of me which I think might prompt someone to spot it, but no.

There is some recognition of change though. People say things like 'you look very well' or they admire my earrings or my dress, but only one picks up that weight is the thing. The truth is that when you're very heavy, a stone or two off isn't really a significant loss. In a way, that allows me to stay in hiding on the issue, which is fine because I'm not ready to talk about it yet. I still fear failure in the end.

It's a lovely party and I'm proud of my brother. He has friends going back many years. Some have travelled a long way for this event and he keeps moving round the room, making sure he spends time with everyone.

My eldest sister Julia is there too, and the plan is that she'll come home to stay overnight with us. When I was a child, she was like a second mother to me. It's lovely to see her and we stay up talking into the small hours with our niece Svetlana, over from New York to spend the Christmas holidays with us in Devon. A rare and precious opportunity for the three of us to be together for a bit.

Like the other guests at the party, my sister has said nothing about my weight loss. I drive her over the moor to catch her train home the morning after the party, I ask if she has noticed I've been on a diet and she says, 'No.'

This is odd. I can understand that people I haven't seen for years might not clock it, but I had thought she would.

'No,' she says, 'I'm afraid I just can't see it, to me you're just my sister. I don't think of you in pounds and ounces.'

A bit crushing, but I take it on the chin. And anyway I'm glad that my weight isn't all she sees.

'I'll probably notice next time I make clothes for you,' she says. She's a dressmaker and has measurements for all of us going back years. With a tape measure in her hand she would have the evidence laid out.

My two sisters and I seemed to have a sort of unwritten deal, roles that we slipped into in childhood. Julia was the beauty, still is. Belinda was the glamorous one, a charmer and a flirt, cool, when I was still a plump bespectacled teenager. I was the clever one. Only this was always nonsense. They were clever as well as pretty. I was bright enough but wasn't a total ugly duckling either. This 'deal' was flawed from the off. But was I forbidden by some unwritten law to change the script and shake up our roles?

I drop her at the station in the pouring rain, water bucketing down our necks as soon as the car door opens. I wave her off, full of love for her departing figure. I don't see enough of her.

But as I drive away I have a sudden thought and start to laugh. 'You really can't see it?' I mutter to myself. 'Really? Just you wait. You will.'

14st 11lbs

Wednesday, 28 December 2011

CHRISTMAS HAS BEEN and gone. I allowed myself three days of total liberty. Three days of eating exactly what I like has a produced exactly what I don't like – nearly three pounds extra. I'm doing my damnedest to get rid of them again before Saturday. That would mean two weeks staying at the same weight over Christmas, a result indeed.

I'm fifty-seven and I'm doing this so that I don't get diabetes like my mother. I'm clear about my objectives, which are specifically health-related. But I can't deny that I love clothes too, and for one of the rare times in my life clothes shopping is becoming a pleasure.

So yes, I'm weathering this Christmas, unlike one ten years ago when disaster struck. I had just come down to live in Devon and was working at ITV. At the beginning of the year I had reached nearly sixteen stone and desperately wanted to lose some weight. I had been to a diet class and between March and December lost about ten pounds. In retrospect, I can't have been trying very hard because that's modest headway, at only a pound lost per month, which is very slow given how heavy I was. By comparison, this year I've dropped nearly three stone in the same amount of time. But still it was something.

I had three weeks off work over the Christmas break and made the staggeringly short-sighted decision to abandon my diet for the whole holiday. You can imagine the rest: by New Year, I had regained every pound it had taken me the previous nine months to lose. And was then so demoralised that I couldn't face starting again and abandoned the diet.

So this New Year is a new page. I'm making slow, slow progress but rejecting the negative and looking for benchmarks to celebrate.

Sobering fact #13: *Holidays seem to increase body weight in adults. Participants seeking to lose weight appeared to increase weight over the holiday period.*

Journal of Obesity, 2017

CHAPTER 14

Bigger because smaller

14st 8lb

Monday, 2 January 2012

Bridget is serene, sitting in the winter sun, gazing at the bare but beautiful landscape.

'Thank you.' I'm almost out of breath, but can't wait to say it.

'I've done it! I'm through Christmas, no harm done.'

She nods and laughs, and I join in.

'Was that your present to me?'

She pats my hand, gently, almost affectionate.

What a thing. To stay the same weight over the biggest food festival of the year feels like a gift from my unconscious.

From time to time it occurs to me that this whole Bridget thing is completely crazy. But then again, it seems to be working so I tell myself, 'Don't knock it.'

BUT JUST AS I relax and congratulate myself on having survived Christmas, it all gets a bit sticky.

Let's just say that self-sabotage is alive and well and living in Devon, in my house. This doesn't mean that Bridget wishes me harm exactly, but the problem is that she doesn't wish me well either. My guess is that she was programmed by patterns learned in early childhood. When stress bites, her default is to return to those patterns and repeat them. I know this. So I resist.

I think of it like the factory setting on a smartphone. My own mental factory settings were a mixed bag with some advantages, it's true, but one particular disadvantage that I'm working hard on right now. I do not want to carry on returning to my old patterns. Can you hear me, Bridget?

Some days are just much harder than others. Some days, like today, I feel hungry all day, I want to graze and let desire lead me where it will in my fridge. That's probably fine for most people, but the problem for me is that I would eat a load of carbs and still never feel full. Not binge exactly, but gradually overload on calories, enough to pile back on those hard-hewn pounds. I'm just not going to do it. So I sit at my desk playing silly online games, dreaming of more productive ways to spend my time, drumming my fingers for distraction. I decide what I'll eat today and then eat it. Sounds so easy, doesn't it?

This is a lonely experience. If I were an alcoholic, I would go to an AA gathering, and share. There would be the fellowship of the meeting, understanding, support. Although weight loss groups are plentiful, I've yet to find one where the underlying issues are honestly and fully expressed. Attending AA meetings over the years with various family members, I've actually envied the rawness of the exchange. Moving stories come up in diet classes too, but only briefly, in among a lot of business that doesn't offer real illumination or insight. Not to me, anyway.

One summer thirty years ago, when I was staying with Crispin in California, I went to a few meetings of Overeaters Anonymous. OA is connected with AA and works on a similar twelve-step programme. The talk in these OA meetings was much richer and more honest than most diet groups I've been to at home but the programme didn't quite resonate with me. The emphasis was on addictive behaviour and although I knew

I had 'issues' with my weight, I was convinced that there was a fundamental difference between them and alcoholism or drug addiction.

There was a lot of focus on recognising the harm done to family, friends and colleagues through addictive behaviour. That makes sense in relation to abuse of alcohol and drugs, but in my view the most damaging aspect of obesity is that it's a form of self-harm. If I needed to make amends to anyone, it was probably myself.

These visits to OA happened many years before I met Chris. When he compared me to an alcoholic, I had a momentary flashback to the stories I had heard in those far off OA meetings, but I quickly put them out of mind. They didn't seem relevant. As you know, I was busy rejecting Chris's analogy with alcoholism out of hand.

How would it feel to give in and eat? There was a time when I would toast a couple of crumpets mid-afternoon, have them with jam and tea. Then maybe a slice of cheese, nuts and a cracker or two. And then perhaps a piece of fruit, a handful of sultanas, another cracker. You see, not quite binging but definitely on course not to lose, maybe even enough to gain a pound or so. I would give in to this desire because I was busy and tired. I felt I could just shut myself up, push away my problems by eating something quickly. It would free me up to pay attention to the rest of the family and to everything else I had to do, all my other responsibilities.

Back to self-sabotage. Definitions include addictions of all sorts – alcoholism, drug misuse, self-harm and overeating. These are negative behaviours, for sure. But 'self-sabotage' is a very loaded phrase, isn't it? There's a ring of judgement about the word sabotage which I'm not sure is useful. It sounds intentional, as if Bridget was sneaking around in a balaclava and black tights, avoiding detection, deliberately undermining my efforts. Maybe that's not it at all.

On the same 'Neuroscience' episode of *In Our Time* as the

discussion about Benjamin Libet, there was an expert in MRI scanning, Gemma Calvert, a professor of applied neuroimaging at Warwick University. She described what happens when you scan the brain of someone who is looking at that famous visual illusion, the black and white silhouette which can be read as either a vase or two faces in profile. As it happens, there are distinct areas in the brain for facial recognition and for objects. She explained that it's not possible to see the image as both face and object at the same time because the brain cells involved are physically separated. You can 'click' between them, but you can't see both simultaneously.

Perhaps the part of the brain that perceives food (alcohol, drugs) as comforting is located in position A and the part that recognises the damage done and the hope of a healthier future is in location B. Then they wouldn't be just emotionally clashing ideas, but physically separated too. Maybe that's why we lurch from one to the other, feasting or fasting, boozing or drying, because we literally can't see both ways forward at the same time. I have no evidence for this idea, but I find it encouraging. It might be why struggling with overeating is so hard and so confusing.

Here's some movement: I do now understand that nothing I eat in this mood will in fact shut me up. Nothing will stop me feeling that I want more. If I allow myself to think what I would like to eat, every one of those snacks, even in imagination, leads to the next. It does not stop the hunger and knowing that changes everything. It means that in this frame of mind there is no point in eating anything. There is only a point in being still, waiting patiently to feel differently.

Remember, two and half pounds a year over forty years is all it took to get where I was when I began.

For supper we have vegetable curry with a very small amount of rice for me, more for the boys. Last time I made this I added a fifty-gram sachet of creamed coconut, which was delicious. Chris asks for the same again. I check the calories – horrendous.

There's the equivalent of a full English breakfast worth of calories in one sachet, no thank you. No can do.

I make a lighter version, followed by a single Viscount biscuit (have cut back here too) and settle down with a cup of black tea to watch telly. Tomorrow will be easier.

14st 7lb

Saturday, 7 January 2012

ANOTHER POUND OFF to welcome in the New Year. I think back to the days when I would start a new diet, gritting my teeth and swearing that this time I wouldn't fall off the wagon, only to slip and slide right away. I'm so glad I'm not there any more.

As we bump along country lanes to a party, I tell Chris I've read that negative thoughts are 'sticky' and hang around in your consciousness doing you harm. You think they act as motivators, but they don't. In fact, they come up like bogeymen in the dark to frighten you. The image they conjure up of the behaviour you're trying to avoid becomes, ironically, a template that you're likely to follow. You don't want to eat the wrong stuff, and thus get or stay overweight, and so you think hard about it. But far from preventing you, this actually puts the idea in your head and makes it more likely to happen. Infuriating.

Chris goes mountain biking across Dartmoor every Thursday evening, all year round, come rain, storm or snow. He says if you're belting downhill and you see a stone you want to avoid, the temptation is to stare at it as you try to steer round it but if you do that, you'll almost certainly hit it. What you need to do is to force your gaze to one side, look at where the path is clear and aim for that, and the bike will go where you're looking. Let the stone take care of itself.

Well that's what I'm doing. Looking at the path ahead, and letting the stones take care of themselves.

14st 6lb

Saturday, 28 January 2012

TODAY I'VE HIT three stone off. Hooray. When I started this thing, I aimed at losing a pound a week. If I had succeeded, I would have reached this point on 4 December, but my way hasn't been quite so smooth. And anyway, date watching of that sort is old think. New think says it can take as long as it likes as long as it keeps on taking.

I went to an awards ceremony last night where I met up with lots of industry colleagues I've known for years but don't bump into very often. Quite suddenly, everyone seemed to notice my new shape. It felt as if I'd come out of the diet closet. Faced with unexpected comment and praise, suddenly I had a great sense of achievement. I felt bigger, all because I was smaller.

A lovely cameraman gave me a sharp nudge in the ribs. 'Nice work. But I don't get it – why didn't you do it years ago? You're powerful enough, why did you need to be bigger?'

He was making the massive and mistaken assumption that people get big to make themselves feel big. I laughed, but this remark struck me between the eyes because it was so much the opposite of what I have ever felt. To be fat in our culture is to be invisible and to say, 'I am no competition. Don't fear me.'

The fat person's prayer goes something like this, 'Please, make me big and then no one will notice me. If you take away the duvet I've wrapped round me all my adult life, I'll have to come out and reveal myself to the world, unprotected. I'll be seen and visible. People (men and women) will react to me, the real me, not the plump cosy packaging I hide inside. I'm not sure that I'm up for it.'

Well now I am up for it. I am not doing it out of competition, but the twin desires of avoiding diabetes and living at peace with Bridget. Not forgetting that I want to wear some nice clothes before I die.

14st 4lb

Saturday, 11 February 2012

'Bridget, I'm going to America for a couple of weeks.'

I'm used to that look. She knows, of course.

'The thing is, I've never come back from America without piling on the pounds. The portions are huge. What do I do?'

She thinks, and raises an eyebrow. I feel as though I can read the answer.

'So you think that I'm on holiday, and any damage I do can be undone as soon as I'm back?'

She nods.

'But you also think I shouldn't go mad ... should use restraint where I can?'

Yes, she nods again, that's about it.

WE FLY TO Los Angeles to visit my brother Crispin. As soon as we walk into his house, he looks me up and down, a big grin all over his face.

'Well look at you!'

The last time I saw him was two years ago in England. We had a memorable car journey together during which he told me he was worried about me because I wasn't 'taking care' of myself. He was obviously talking about my weight. At the time I was busy protecting my own (inert) position on obesity, and it made me furious. I said nothing, because I love him and don't see him often enough to fight with him when I do. Instead, I drummed my fingers on the dashboard in silent fury, willing him to shut up and leave me alone. Eventually he did.

Now it's different. I can tell he's pleased and proud, and that he understands I've been fighting demons to get where I am. Of my mother's six children, I'm the only one to have inherited her massive weight problem. Why is that? I don't know, but some of the others have struggled with alcohol or drugs and Belinda was a yo-yo dieter, though never reaching the extremes that I did. We are obviously an addictive lot.

Personally, I hardly drink at all, not for any particular reason that I'm aware of, except that I just can't do it. I avoid spirits, rarely drink beer, and take only an occasional glass of wine. Sometimes I throw caution to the wind and accept a second glass, but inevitably find that I don't touch it. I've long since believed that my sensitivity to it is like a kind of inverted alcoholism – as if the same genes that have made one or two of my siblings susceptible have made me mildly intolerant.

LA IS A wonderful city to visit when you know people who live there. We go on an unofficial tour of Frank Gehry architecture, visit the Getty museum and Venice Beach. My brother takes us to his favourite restaurants: a Mexican on the corner near his home for a rich, dark chocolate mole, and a Korean nearby for noodles and meatballs. He also cooks us fabulous food at home.

Orlando's favourite part of the whole trip is the day we go to a diner. I know already what I'm going to eat: American pancakes with maple syrup. I had fantasised about this wicked delight before I even got to the US and decided to just go with it. They're delicious – kind of – but before I've even finished them I am already thinking, 'I can live without these again for a year or two.' Just as well.

If I was an alcoholic I would never be in this position, of taking a hit and then deciding not to do it again for a year. We would all know that one slip could, probably would, lead to a massive slide. But with food it's different, you can't give it up. There's a never-ending series of opportunities to make good or bad choices, to be firm or falter, to test yourself and either win through or find yourself wanting.

Given that problem, the issue of making and breaking food resolutions goes to the heart of the matter. Perhaps we dieters distort our own ability to exercise self-control by constantly fighting our own desires, and then losing the battle. I won't – I'm not going to – I could just – might as well – oh look I've done it – no point holding back now. We get used to being on a losing streak, losing against our own better judgement.

Learning to give yourself positive permission to eat seems to me just as important as learning to resist. If you really want a particular food – go for it. Eat it with relish, whole-heartedly, without self-judgement. Mindfully. Then, if necessary, use restraint later on. That's the spirit in which I ate those American pancakes. Play then pay.

Earlier on in this project, I wouldn't have done this. At that time, I was learning to practise restraint in a sustained way. But here I am, on holiday, with a three stone weight loss behind me, deciding to relax for a short while. It's fine.

I imagine I'm on a high wire, finding my balance and walking on over. At worst, as if I might slip at any time, with terrible consequences. At best, as if I've found my centre and am holding it.

Sobering fact #14: *It is difficult to maintain weight loss. Contestants on The Biggest Loser lost an average of 127lb each but over time thirteen of fourteen gained 66 per cent of the weight lost.*

Obesity, 2016
Time, 2017

CHAPTER 15

Not mindful but fearful

14st 8lb

Saturday, 18 February 2012

'Bridget – four pounds on. What do you think?'

What did I expect her to say? Could have been better, could have been worse? She doesn't give much away.

And then I realise that the real test is not what happened in America, but what happens next.

'How long to do you think it'll take to put it right?'

She gives me a straight look. OK, I get it, wrong question.

'So it doesn't matter how long it takes, I should just get back on that horse and get trucking?'

She nods, picks up her wheelbarrow, and trundles off. Me too. I can take a hint.

CLEAR AND FOCUSED, I'm ready for the next onslaught and talking up the motivation. I picture dieting as a battleground and cast myself as my own sergeant major, barking instructions to myself.

When you stand in front of an aisle full of chocolate, or biscuits, or cake – whatever it is that tempts you ... and you dither, and pick up a bar of chocolate, put it back, take a Milky Way because it's smaller, put it back, reach out again, pull back, turn round and walk away – that's when you're on the front line in the battle of the bulge.

You may be ashamed that this struggle ever comes your way, and wish you could deny that it happens, but you know it does. Far from a moment of shame, this is the moment for your courage to rise, and your adrenaline to surge – this is when you're in the heat of battle.

These are the stages:

1. Deciding to diet is strategy formation – you're in the War Room. The generals are gathering, considering how to mobilise.
2. Picking a diet regime is arming up – you're equipping yourself with the means to fight. This is the technical bit. Now you have the tools you need to do battle.
3. This is the frontline of the war on weight: standing helpless, tempted and confused, listening to the voices in your head that tell you one more slip will make no difference, resisting anyway. This is where it's won or lost, despite what those voices say.

The problem is that it's humiliating to confess that this happens, embarrassing to admit that it's so hard to stay firm and mortifying when you can't. This is the moment when you are tested. It's the moment when you are at the heart of the problem.

Every one of the minor victories helps you on your way. Your inner voice will no doubt (like mine) be rabbiting on at you, telling you that resisting temptation this once is nothing, won't help, won't get you anywhere, is a waste of effort. But it's not true. Simple logic tells you that every time you give in, you repeat old patterns you want to be shot of. Every time you resist, you're improving your chances.

13st 13lb

Saturday, 17 March 2012

IT'S CLEARER ALL the time that finding Bridget was the key strategy in my battle to lose weight, more important that I knew when I started out. I needed a way to look past the obvious, to find something between mediation and reflection that would help me get to the truth of the matter.

I wanted to send my unconscious a message in a bottle, hoping it would land. That's the best we can do, words alone are not it.

To contact her is easy. The best analogy is a stereogram, a 2D image in a seemingly random pattern which, if you defocus your eyes in a particular way, reveals a hidden 3D object. Stereograms were briefly fashionable in the eighties. At first I found them frustrating because, however hard I tried, I couldn't see the hidden shark, or bunch of flowers, or scorpion, which everyone else said they could. When I finally managed it, I was mesmerised. A blur of coloured dots gradually resolved into an underwater scene, with coral, plankton and a school of swooping fish. I gazed and gazed, feeling as if I had entered that underwater world.

To get there, I had to learn to look into the distance even with a page up close in front of me. That's what it's like to contact Bridget. She's distant, but up close. She's always there, but I can't always see her. Her meaning is clear, but I can't always receive it. Her message seems to be emotional, rather than rational.

According to Kahneman, the brain's 'system 1' is not much good at solving hard cognitive problems like long division, planning ahead or translating complex sentences into another language. Since Bridget resembles 'system 1' quite closely, I begin to wonder how she would fare if set those sorts of problems. I climb up to her eyrie to test this out with an experiment.

Bridget's perched on a rock, gazing at the horizon, when I arrive.

I hand her a Rubik's cube, the colours all jumbled. She looks at it with some distaste.

'Can you do it?' I ask.

She takes it from me, twisting and turning it, fast, this way and that, impatient. She's doesn't seem to be getting anywhere.

Suddenly, she hands it back to me. It feels odd. Is she asking for help? No, she's imperious. She's delegating.

'I'll give it a go,' I say. She nods.

I twist it a few times and move it on. All the greens are lining up nicely.

She raises an eyebrow. Cognitive work is obviously a waste of her talents. It's not what she's for. She sheds light on so much but in this department, Kahneman seems to be right – I'm on my own.

I TALK TO Sarah, funny and practical business affairs manager in a neighbouring television company. I've known her for a long time. I suppose she's always been a little rounded, but she has marvellous cheekbones which cover a multitude of sins. But from the odd rushed conversation in corners over the years, I know she struggles with her weight.

From what I can see she's never been more than a couple of stone overweight, nursery slopes compared to me. She took six months maternity leave after the births of each of her children, and after the third came back to work much slimmer. She'd been to a diet class and shed all her baby weight and then some. Gradually a bit of excess has crept back on and now she's trying to lose again.

Like me, she knows without having to think too hard how heavy she was at every milestone of her adult life. That's not a good thing, by the way, but a sign of having been constantly stressed by the subject. Her problems began as a teenager. Her mum, like mine, had always been very overweight and was constantly dieting. Once she reached her early twenties, it seemed natural for Sarah to go with her to a diet class. She's been on a weight see-saw ever since. She describes it as a permanent anxiety and later in the day sends me a link to a song that whistles through her brain all the time – 'It's hard to dance with the devil on your back – so shake him off!'

My weight loss has opened up the subject. People who once wouldn't have dreamed of sharing their adventures in the food minefield now often do it. Sometimes they have a hungry look, as though I have a magic bullet I could give them, if only I would. I prefer that to the ones who get competitive. That's not pretty, and leaves me perplexed.

This week I had meetings in London and found time in the middle for lunch with Carol, an old friend I hadn't seen for a year. As I walked across the restaurant to meet her, she didn't quite recognise me, and then did a double take and realised it was me. She was bowled over, says being thinner makes me look younger. She's another fellow traveller, and tells me she's put on a stone since we last met.

She was desperate to know how I've done it, eyes alive with interest. It feels like there's too much to tell. 'It's a trick of the mind,' I say, which seems the closest thing to the truth. It's what I've taken to saying when I'm asked.

Sometimes I think people are more satisfied if I just say Weight Watchers. 'Oh Weight Watchers!' they say, as if that explains it. But as you know that's the tip of the iceberg. The diet, yes, the frame of mind, no.

She kept asking for more details and so I described my Cadover Bridge moment. She got it completely. She tells me that she often eats in a comatose sort of way, getting through huge platefuls while barely tasting what's in her mouth. There was something wistful in the way she talked, as though she feels change is hopelessly out of reach.

We both ordered salmon and broccoli, delicious. She had chips on the side with mayonnaise and gestured to me to help myself. I had a couple. Then, without asking, she ordered a tarte tatin for us to share. When it arrived, she cut it square down the middle. For sociability I had a couple of spoonfuls. This was not for show, but because I had made a deal with myself and was sticking to it. She ate exactly her half and no more. She said she isn't on a diet but seemed to be holding back, silently urging me to finish 'my' bit (not ordered by me). Not mindful, but fearful.

Memories of my mother's desire to recruit me into her fat fest spring immediately to mind, as well as her reaction, crushed disappointment whenever I managed to hold off.

I'd like to find a way of saying to Carol, and others, quite clearly, 'no provocation intended'. It's hard enough for me to stick to my plan, even harder when, from other people's reactions, I sense that it reads as a challenge.

I am keeping myself in balance, doing what I'd planned to do. Not out of competition, but out of respect and love for Bridget, who is I think quite happy at the moment.

13st 13lb

Monday, 26 March 2012

THEN BANG – on Saturday I had a feeding frenzy, probably the worst since I began to diet. I ate the first packet of crisps I've had for eight months (not that good, I was glad to find), a packet of Revels (still great), a baked potato, a piece of bread ... I felt completely out of control.

Actually, now I come to think of it, I see that it wasn't as bad as it felt. One of the problems with us body dysmorphics is that we have little sense of proportion when it comes to food. Sometimes it feels like we've had a total blow out and it was actually a small indulgence. Sometimes it's the opposite: we're in denial, having consumed a ton of food that we've carefully forgotten about.

I try to be rigorous about writing everything down, track it even if I have to guess quantities or ingredients when I eat away from home. The simple act of remembering and recording is helpful. It keeps me mindful.

There is a counter-argument here though: writing every-thing down feels over-controlled, as if I'm fixating on it, and in turn that might be feeding my obsessive behaviour around food. This is such a minefield. I need to lose weight to get healthy. I want to rid myself of food obsession. How do those things work together? I'm still trying to understand.

I decide to visit Bridget, hoping to connect with her, and perhaps come to some compromise about how to act in this crazy state of mind. This is based on the assumption that she's guiding my actions even if I can't understand her reasoning.

Except of course in the past I've left this situation to her and haven't always been impressed with the outcome, viz. ending up seven stone overweight. Just saying.

Bridget could tell me what's going on – but she isn't playing. I don't even get as far as her cave. It is clear on approach that she isn't feeling receptive. Sometimes when she's bent on chaos we get a bit of radio silence before she comes back online.

I think hard and send her a message. 'What's happening? Am I losing it?'

Silence.

'Will I be able to get back on track tomorrow?'

Silence.

'What if I can't? Should I keep my old clothes just in case?'

Silence of such black depth that I finally get the message – there's not going to be an answer tonight. With which I have to be content.

HERE'S ANOTHER WAY to think about self-sabotage. Bridget is a quick thinker, intuitive and visual, who seeks out patterns and associations. She is preoccupied with scanning for possible dangers and taking evasive action as necessary. When faced with temptation, all she sees is instant gratification. She doesn't look at history or repercussions. She has no reason not to give in.

I – that, is my verbalising, planning ahead, talking to myself I – I am more like Kahneman's 'system 2', slow, cognitive and methodical. I am the record-keeper of past events and the future planner. I can remember the pain caused by overeating and want to avoid reproducing that pain in the future. When faced with temptation, I can see plenty of reasons to resist.

The problem is that Bridget rules. She's faster, so she gets in first. She's in charge of everything from motor function to stress management. Her decisions precede mine. She wins.

Except not always. We can reprocess. We can rethink. We can hold our own prejudices and assumptions up to the light and re-examine them, see if they fit our adult beliefs. If that isn't true, then there really is no hope of change.

BETWEEN SCHOOL AND university I travelled overland to India. I caught a bus one day at Totteridge Tube station in London, and four weeks later we motored through the Khyber Pass into Pakistan. Then, travelling by local buses and trains, I roamed around India and Nepal, revisiting places my mother lived in as a child. I retraced her steps, mapping her early family life, when she moved between Delhi and Peshawar, and then moved up to the hill station in Simla (now Shimla) for the summer to escape the heat of the plains.

Most of the people I met on the bus got ill, suffering dysentery and severe weight loss at one stop or another. Not me. Whenever I was concerned about food hygiene (often, as this was budget travel) I stuck to dal and rice, with an occasional foray into sag paneer or naan. I avoided most meat and all fish.

Occasionally there was a so-called English breakfast on offer, with thin soft toast like savoury brioche, fried eggs and sauté potatoes with cumin. But mostly I lived on dal. I was rarely hungry, buoyed by a huge sense of excitement at being on my own, entirely responsible for myself for the first time and in a position to reinvent myself, post-childhood, in this new group of people.

The result was that I came home a couple of stone lighter, not from illness but from this very simple food, eating modestly, happily absorbed in my new experiences. Back in the UK, there was still a month to go before I was due to start university. I headed straight up to Scotland to join my mother, who was cooking at a grand house party where there was a grouse shoot. She got me a job as a housemaid. The work was drudgery and required both punctuality and deference. I wasn't good at either. But it was a rare opportunity to spend a solid stretch of time with her. She remained elusive, hard to pin down, absent even though right there, stuck in the middle of the Scottish Highlands with me.

Sometimes I think it's because I don't understand her that she still occupies my imagination. I think of her often, and wonder what made her tick.

And wonder, too, whether the newly slimmed down version of me that stepped off the train at Pitlochry was a challenge to her.

'Well, look at you!' she said, taking me in, her words strangely foreshadowing Crispin's reaction thirty-five years later in Los Angeles.

AT WORK, ANNA asked me today what the secret of my new-found success is. I suppose it's getting more obvious that I really am doing it – three stone gone. I tell her about mindfulness. I describe what I'm reading about the unconscious, about it not being a dark and fearful enemy but a part of our mind which works to a different rhythm, responding to stimuli in quite another way. I tell her about the white noise in my head which is the verbal self, wittering on, full of words and phrases, signifying nothing, constantly telling me it won't work and can't be done. She keeps encouraging me to go on.

In the end, a little self-consciously, I tell her about Bridget. Anna's a bit of a cynic and I'm nervous about her reaction, but she gets the idea right away.

'Anastasia,' she says.

'Ah, so you have an Anastasia?'

She tells me that her jeans get tighter, and she worries about it, but can't control it. In the evenings she often finds herself on the sofa with a biscuit in her hand.

'There you are. That's what I'm talking about. That's the Cadover Bridge Syndrome. Well, I think you and Anastasia need to communicate.'

'But the trouble is you do sound a bit mad,' she says. 'Zealous.'

I'm sure I do.

13st 12lb

Monday, 9 April 2012

'MUM, WHAT DO you weigh?' Orlando has asked this me over and over again since I began this long trek through the diet wilderness.

'I've told you before – I'm not telling you.'

Chris chips in. 'Didn't you say you'd tell us when you're lighter than me?'

I did. And I am – but hadn't even noticed that I've passed another benchmark.

'What are you, hon? Fourteen stone?'

'Yes.'

'And you?' to Orlando.

'No, wait a minute – he wasn't part of it.'

'Just over fourteen.'

They both look hard at me.

'You must be getting close,' Chris says.

'Aagh. You're right – but I find it really hard to say ... 13st 12lb! There. Done it.'

ALCOHOLICS ANONYMOUS IS a lifeline for millions and I have huge respect for the programme, but I do have one issue with it. As part of the twelve-step programme, six of the steps mention God 'as we understood him'. In the programme, God is often referred to as a 'Higher Power' which I assume is intended to universalise the message so that people of any religion feel able subscribe to it.

Personally, I've always found the notion troublesome. It suggests some kind of submission to an outside force, which doesn't resonate with me. But it occurs to me to wonder – is Bridget my Higher Power? I don't think so. In my mind there's nothing ethereal or spiritual about her. She's just a hidden part of me.

Every day I think this is all a big con. Yes, I lost three stone before Christmas, but I've hardly moved an inch since then. I feel like a fraud when people say I'm still shedding pounds because I know I'm not. I'm aware how slow it is and how many battles I still face. But just now I looked back to my record and three months ago, I was nine pounds heavier than I am this week. This diet can take as long as it likes. It's going to work.

13st 10lb

Friday, 20 April 2012

TODAY WE'RE EATING in a local pub, a dozen of us, very sociable. We live near a big local hospital and many of our neighbours and friends are medics of one sort or another. A few years ago, we were having supper in this same group which included three doctors. Statins were new on the market and one them asked me, as small talk really, whether I would consider taking a pill a day on the off chance that it would prevent me from having heart disease or a stroke.

'Don't think so,' I was glib. 'Anyway, I'm not planning on a stroke. Diabetes is more my style.'

I meant to be funny but no one laughed. The particular quality of the small silence that followed was not lost on me. My friends are kind, and they'll probably deny it, but Type 2 diabetes might as well have been written in neon on their foreheads.

Back to tonight's dinner. I take the food order to the bar. On Fridays I am always rigorous, the looming Saturday morning weigh-in keeping me on track. There is a moment of fear as I am about to be served – what will I order for myself? I am actually scared of what I will say. I run through eleven meals, and get to my own. I think of Bridget.

'And a chicken Caesar salad, please.' As soon as I've ordered, anguish over. Decision made, triumph for me and Bridget. Done.

I am a middle-aged woman with an imaginary friend. Get over it.

Sobering fact #15: *In the UK, we spend over £11 billion a year on care of Type 2 diabetes and its complications.*

LSE Health, 2012

CHAPTER 16

My imaginary friend disappears

13st 9lb

Friday, 27 April 2012

I toil up the hillside again. I soon find myself at Bridget's cave and there are a few smouldering remains of her fire, but no sign of her. I root around for a bit, hoping she'll turn up, but then the sound of branches cracking in the distance tells me where she is – doing a bit of tree work, from the sounds of it.

Immediately I realise that I shouldn't follow her into the woods. She doesn't want me to. It would be overdramatic to say that she's avoiding me, but there's a definite sense of reluctance. Why?

Sometimes I really wish she'd speak. It would be so much easier than this crazy puzzling, trying to work out what she thinks, and whether she's trying to tell me something. Of course, she isn't. She isn't trying to communicate with me at all. She's quite content to carry on just as she is. It's me that wants to change.

So this time I have to think hard about what might be going on. I can see two distinct possibilities: either she's bent on more bad behaviour, eating-wise, and doesn't want to discuss it because she doesn't want to stop; or she's got some hidden agenda which she thinks is for my benefit. Maybe she even thinks she's protecting me.

I don't like any of these scenarios. Objectively speaking, losing weight is a good thing. It's benefiting my health, I feel more comfortable in my clothes and I like the positive feedback I'm getting. Therefore I think she may be mistaken – please note the respectful tone. But how to get her to see that? We're on dangerous ground here because I know – and this is where I began this journey – that I can't lecture her into submission.

I want to say to her, 'Do you realise that my odds of developing Type 2 diabetes are three to one if I remain obese?' But as I know that, so does she. Obviously.

I poke around in the cave for a bit, hoping she'll return. She doesn't. Eventually I make my way disconsolately back down the hill back to reality. She isn't coming out to play today. That means I have even less of a clue than usual about her attitude to my diet. Will she sabotage it, and leave me struggling out of control? I'll just have to wait and see.

IN FACT WHAT happens is that I have a reasonable supper plus some unreasonable pudding (bananas and custard, delicious), go to bed and rise, resolute once again. Two days on and I'm back in the programme, relieved and grateful – yes, grateful to Bridget for not making it harder than it already is. She's the boss of me, and she seems to be letting me do it.

'MUM, HOW MANY calories should I be eating for lunch?'

I'm torn by this question. Pleased that he's considering it, anxious that he doesn't obsess. At fifteen he shouldn't be worrying about his weight, but on the other hand information is power. It occurs to me that I might be more anxious about this conversation if he were a girl because of the fear of anorexia. But in this case, a bit of level-headed advice won't come amiss.

'At your height you should be aiming at about 2500 calories a day. So maybe six or seven hundred or so for lunch.'

'So is a whole packet of Pringles bad?'

'Almost certainly. Look it up.'

'Wow. That's over a thousand.'

'... almost entirely made up of fat and sugar. There's your answer then.'

WHAT DO NEGATIVE feelings feel like? A sick sensation in the lower abdomen, heavy shoulders, tiredness, nail biting, pursed mouth.

I'm gutted because my colleague Lauren is leaving work. I'm not sleeping well, am miserable, and to cap it all, permanently slightly hungry. I'm committed to my diet and still clear that I don't want to abandon it. But some part of the brain (not Bridget this time) tells me that if I eat a lot of sugar and fat I'll feel better.

Luckily my verbal self and Bridget are united on this point. We think it'll make me feel much worse. And of course it would. Added to the feelings of loss and disappointment on the colleague front would be a sense of failure with the diet. The short-term lift from the food would be followed by no weight loss tomorrow, maybe even a gain that would take another week or so to undo. It's not even a battlefield. I'm at a point where I know what I have to do and there's just no reason not to do it. But that nagging sensation of gnawing hunger grumbles away at me, making it harder than ever to pick myself up. Writing is a sort of therapy.

I sit here trying to be truthful about what's happening to me. On the positive side, every day this week I've felt a little trimmer. From experience I know that's a good sign and means I'm likely to lose again this week. At the same time I feel a little vulnerable, blowing about like a reed in the wind. I want this, but the body is programmed to maintain itself as the same level and so of course feels under pressure when it's gradually shrinking.

Losing weight feels like the tide going out. If you watch it you can barely see the movement, but if you look away for half an hour, it's made a jump.

Why should I be so sad about a colleague leaving work? Because she's brilliant, makes me laugh, keeps everyone focused and brings in new work. But most of all because I'll miss her: playing Scrabble on our endless trips to London, racing to finish Codeword, gossiping, squabbling and testing out new ideas.

But people have to do what they have to do. It feels like the end of something glorious, but of course it could just be that I fear change. I'll have to move on too.

ONE DAY IN the office everyone is chatting and the subject of flashing crops up. It turns out Gilly has been flashed many times. Our male colleagues are horrified to hear this but the women are resigned. Things like that have happened to everyone. Gilly says she knew someone who was even flashed walking across Hampstead Heath in broad daylight.

A sudden flashback to a flasher of my own, coincidentally in the same place. I am ten and a man in a black cashmere coat approaches me as I cross the heath on my way home from school. He says he is a plain clothes policeman and tells me that there is someone dodgy around, bothering young girls. He asks if I've seen anyone like that.

'No, I haven't.'

'Let me show you what he does.' He leads me under the trees.

'Sit here next to me. That's right. Now this man – let me show you and then you'll know what to look out for.' He pushes me onto my back on the ground.

The scent of the grass, newly cut, the shade of a huge sweeping chestnut tree. Hidden from view. The sound of children yelling as they sail boats on Whitestone Pond. Passers-by, heels clicking on tarmac in the distance.

'He'll push you back like this, and then this is what he'll do ...'

I suddenly realise that something is very wrong. I jump to my feet.

'I have to go,' I blurt out and dash away, running like crazy across the wide open grassland, heart hammering, not daring to look back, towards my mother who works half a mile away.

She laughs when I tell her. 'You were clever. You saw him off.' But still she phones the police.

Who was this man? I don't know. He told me he was a policeman and I believed him. It was only when he pushed me down on the grass that it suddenly felt wrong. What did he do? Nothing, I ran away.

I consider adding my bit to the office banter, but Gilly is so vocal, insistent and emphatic that everyone is caught up in the drama. I realise I can't make light of it, so I don't.

13st 8lb

Friday, 18 May 2012

ANOTHER PLATEAU, ANOTHER challenge to belief. The noise in my mind today whispers on that this is fruitless, bootless, hopeless and will never work. But this of course is familiar territory. A little shaft of hope forces its way through: it will work, it can't not work, there is no reason to stop, the rewards are great and persistence is fruitful.

Last weekend I went to a reunion in Bristol and met up with an ex-colleague from years back, called Alex. We were researchers together in our twenties and since then her career has gone stellar. She's a very clever woman who may one day run one of our major television channels. Over the last five years she's lost nearly seven stone. She patted her size 10 stomach and murmured that she's half a stone heavier than she should be. Chorus of approval all round. You look fantastic (she does), like a model (she does).

Every time I see her she talks about her weight. She mentions that she's still not thin enough, and draws attention to some allegedly failing part of her anatomy with the result that everyone looks at it – and admires. Has she ever acknowledged that I've lost anything at all? You bet your sweet ass she hasn't.

To be fair I'm still a generous size 16, but I'm pretty sure it's a transformation. It makes me smile but only on the inside. The point is that it can't hurt me because Bridget is on my side and that's all I need. I'm in the normal sphere now and everything from here on is moving me towards a healthy weight.

People's reactions are amazing, complicated and compromised. Soon I'm anticipating that someone will be taking me to one side and saying they're worried about me and that I'm going too far, losing too much. I predict that'll happen in about a stone from now. By then I'll be 12st 7lb, and still substantially overweight. I don't think that'll stop them.

I say again, people's reactions are extraordinary. My great friend Rosie has been a big support to me. She was diagnosed with high blood pressure at the beginning of last year and started to do serious amounts of exercise. She made a habit of going to the gym before work four times a week. Soon her weight began to drop and now, two stone off, she looks fabulous.

She met up with our mutual friend Carol recently who, like Alex with me, completely blanked her weight loss. Rosie came away miserable and furious in equal measure, determined to 'have it out with her' and let her know how hurt she felt. I understand, of course, but don't feel the same way. I think people do those things because of the battles inside their own heads. Having had plenty of battles of my own, I have some sympathy with the blankers. It's tough out here – for everyone concerned.

But much more significantly, I feel protected. I'm beating to a different drum. This is all about me and Bridget. I'm so busy making peace with her and trying to negotiate a harmonious way forward in my own mind, I don't have time to worry about other people's reactions, which is frankly a relief.

Judgement seems to lie all around. There's an implicit criticism from some people, which I sense, although it's never quite articulated: why do you want to lose weight anyway – vanity? You're too old for it to matter. But on this I have complete clarity. I am losing weight because I don't want to get Type 2 diabetes. And also I like new dresses.

Our relationship with weight is such a mess. Obsession with dieting is dangerous and life denying, anti-feminist and sad. And yet being seriously overweight is all those things too. We should not have to retreat into protecting ourselves from female competition, the full experience of our own feelings or unwanted sexual attention by becoming overweight. That's not female empowerment but subjugation of a whole different sort. How is anyone supposed to adopt a rational approach to all this? The answer is to find a healthy weight to aim for, get there and stay there. However, that's not straightforward, as we know.

I have a favourite line from *Absolutely Fabulous* on this very topic. Edina rages about the constant need to diet, the pressure to be slim. 'When will we ever be thin enough?' she asks. 'When? A few moments after death – is that it?'

Anyway, back to Carol, Rosie's and my friend. She's also overweight, probably obese, although of course we would never name it as that. Were we drawn together as friends because we all had weight issues? I don't think so. It feels like a coincidence, but I'm not sure. Anyway, Carol rang me about a week ago to catch up. She mentioned that she'd seen Rosie, and said how 'well' she looks. This is code for 'has shed a bit'. Why do we need a code? I really don't know. Carol has avoided the subject of weight loss with Rosie for months now but, following my lunch with her, she's become a bit more straightforward with me. This time she asks me right out how my own campaign is going. I am offhand but truthful.

'Still trundling along, chipping away,' I say.

She asked how much I've lost now. 'Three and half stone,' I say.

'Well done you,' and I heard a particular metallic ring, a kind of mechanical echo in her voice, 'and what about Rosie?'

'I'm not sure, but not far behind I think.'

It's as if she's forcing herself to ask. She's not enthusiastic. I don't take this as a judgement of me or Rosie, but as a sign of her own pain around this issue. While her weight steadily climbs, and both of ours drop, it begs the question of what is happening to her. If we lose more and she carries on gaining, it's seems like a betrayal, as if she's abandoned. She may want to wish us well but there are too many echoes for her.

Sobering fact #16. *An analysis of 57,000 women in 2013 found that those who experienced physical or sexual abuse as children were twice as likely to be addicted to food than those who did not.*

Obesity, 2013

CHAPTER 17

No reason not to succeed ...

13st 6lb

Saturday, 9 June 2012

'Bridget – who's in charge? You or me?' She gives me a level look.

'I've assumed it's you. I'm deferring to you. Is that right?'

She clasps her hands around her knees and stares into the fire. If only she spoke she'd be a great storyteller – she holds all my attention, and I hang on her every gesture. But there's no hint of an answer.

'I need to know whether I should be doing more. Should I be trying to help you work it all out?'

Like an anxious, twittering C-3Po to her mega-brained R2-D2, I'm fretting and fuming while she just sits there, beeping and whistling.

I'll say this for myself – I do try. She doesn't seem inclined to join in. I'm beginning to see that change isn't her thing. She seems to like the status quo.

She stirs the fire, and gazes into the approaching twilight, where the moon has already risen, a pale crescent against a deep blue sky. I sense that I've lost her attention.

The conversation, such as it was, is over.

I'M CELEBRATING A year at this particular coalface on Monday. If you remember, I committed to diet for a year. I had six stone to lose (plus a few stray pounds we don't talk about). I've lost nearly four stone. The question of whether I'll carry on doesn't even arise. I've got the bit between my teeth. Even more important, I've learned to believe that change is possible. I can't say that clearly enough. I spent years suffering doubt and defeat, and now I believe that change is possible. It is possible. It is actually happening.

To break through the latest plateau I've been super rigorous this week and finally some more weight is shifting. I'm keeping it up until Tuesday next week when we're going out to dinner with Molly and Jim, which will officially be a no-holds-barred experience. There's no point eating in a Michelin-starred restaurant and counting points. Having said that, we know they will serve tiny portions with great intensity of flavour.

Orlando is coming, despite some understandable reservations about spending an evening with four adults. Also, being vegetarian, he is used to the utter predictability of eating out menus: cheese salad, mushroom tagliatelle or an omelette. I promise him that both the dishes and the company will be more interesting than he fears.

He's a foodie, like me, and in the past has been a major carb-head. Over the last few months he has gradually fined down, shooting up in height without adding pounds. The day I notice this I see an article in the *Daily Mail* declaring that the best way to help your child lose weight is to lose it yourself. No one knows whether that's role modelling or the result of changes to the family diet, but it seems to be consistent.

Orlando says it's coincidence, but then he would. Either way, it's a great result. We talk about my weight loss on the way home tonight. He tells me how proud he is of me. I tell him I'm worried I'll never get to my goal of a BMI of 25.

'Yes you will. I would literally bet my life on it,' he says. 'I think you'll get to a weight you're happy at and stay there.' I'm taken aback by his certainty.

'I can't see how you would not. Why wouldn't you? You know how to do it. You don't have any reason not to succeed.'

I love the uncompromising clarity of his fourteen-year-old point of view. It's so encouraging to hear him cheer me on like that but it's also a responsibility. I told him I would do it and I wanted to show him it's possible. So now I have to follow through.

13st 5lb

Saturday, 16 June 2012

I'VE HAD A very blue day. We failed to get a contract for a programme which was to be an exploration of food and art. We're all scratchy and disappointed. It was a late cancellation – all dates booked months since, great talent lined up, just waiting for the greenlight that never came.

I'm upset, but I'm not eating my way out of trouble, because of course that would be eating my way into trouble. The short-term solution of old was to pop into the garage on the way home from work for a bag of crisps and a small chocolate bar before supper.

Why both crisps and chocolate? I prefer savoury, but then a mouthful of something sweet to follow always feels right, like a mini meal. Probably the same number of calories as a mini meal too. Not any more.

13st 5lb

Saturday, 23 June 2012

OUR FINE DINING treat was fabulous and Orlando loved it. All four of us adults could see that it was a complete culinary awakening for him: food as an art form. Far from being short-changed, his vegetarian meal was amazing. He had never had such an elaborate series of intensely flavoured dishes in one sitting.

'It's a feast. They haven't put a foot wrong.' Chris loves our rare visits to this great restaurant as much as I do.

'This is the first time I've tasted cooking that makes yours look bad,' says Orlando, with teenage wit.

'I'm glad you like it. Now get a job which lets you eat like this sometimes when you're grown up.' Tit for tat.

WHILE I WAS still at school I developed my taste for really good restaurants. My mother and I would traipse around the Somerset countryside, London, Bristol or Bath, looking for places which were well-reviewed to try out. Restaurant food in Britain at that time was poverty stricken, lazy and unimaginative so it took some searching to find creative cooking. By chance, we were lucky enough to stumble across the Hole in the Wall in Bath and were so impressed that it quickly became our favourite.

The Hole in the Wall was exceptional. Everything was made from scratch, from the breadsticks before the meal to the petits fours served with coffee. That's not unusual these days but in 1970 it was radical. They served roasted onions with herb butter. *Aïoli*, that taste of my childhood. Salmon en croute. Handmade fudge and nougat. Although it wasn't easy to get to and we couldn't really afford it, we went time and again.

Years later, I discovered that the Hole in the Wall's founder, George Perry-Smith, was one of the great names of post-war cooking in Britain. I was very lucky to meet him and enjoy his incredible work, very lucky that my mother appreciated it too.

This whole business of food is so mixed up between positive and negative, pleasure and pain, conflict and harmony.

*

A COMPOSER WE often work with came in to see me today. I last saw Phil before Christmas, although we've spoken on the phone frequently since then. He looked confused.

'Have you lost weight?'

'Yes – nearly four stone.'

'Since when?'

'Last June – so you saw me several times during the first six months. Then there's been a gap and suddenly it's obvious.'

'Well you look great on it.'

We spend some time discussing the music on one of our new shows, and wandering into areas we don't usually discuss – the feast or famine nature of production – rebranding – our own perception of what we're doing and where we are going.

Every now and then he looked at me quizzically, as if reassessing me. After ten years of working together, I can't really believe weight loss has changed his impression of me so much. It was just fat. I haven't had a personality change.

On leaving he leans forward slightly as if to kiss me goodbye. We never do that, so I'm taken aback. It's kindly, complimentary, as though my achievement needs marking; nice but a bit odd. What passes through my mind is, 'This is still me. I'm the same person.'

I can't quite compute the subtle change in the atmosphere but it's definitely positive.

13st 5lb

Thursday, 28 June 2012

YESTERDAY CHRIS SET off on an epic cycle ride from Land's End to John O'Groats. Today he passes through Devon and so comes home for the night, a perfect opportunity to pick up everything he's forgotten (contact lenses, sun cream, more shorts) before setting off again, this time for two and half weeks away. He also gets to say hello and goodbye to Orlando, just back from a school trip to Paris.

A lovely evening. I cooked favourite suppers for my boys, big and small, as a goodbye for now: steak and mushrooms for Chris, Quorn and tarragon pie for Orlando, my special apple crumble for both of them. We bounce round the kitchen, jigging along to Jack Johnson, happy to be back together for one more evening before another separation.

Just before bed I get a furious email from one of our presenters. We're due to film with him for fifteen days from Sunday. He's just read through the filming call sheet and is objecting to the plans. Bad weather has given us some script problems and we have a solution, in my view the only practical one, but he doesn't agree and hasn't been available for the past ten days to discuss it. I've written at length explaining why we should do it this way but he's adamant that we've got it all wrong.

Meanwhile, unable to talk it through with him, we have had to press ahead. We've produced a twenty-seven-page call sheet with detailed arrangements on every line involving crew and contributors, health and safety, transport and script for the next two weeks. At this late stage, a radical change of plan would be very difficult to implement. As I try to think how I can explain, briefly because I know how busy he is, but really clearly, so there will be no further argument, I am breathless. Chris makes sensible suggestions but he can see that I am very stressed.

I draft a reply but don't send it. We go to bed. I keep waking up, trivial details of the shoot coursing through my brain … must remember to put the lemon curd on the bus … where are those porcelain coffee cups … do the crew realise they have to motor from A to B in the break … there's only a two-hour window … what if they don't make it … I don't cry but I bite my nails, toss and turn, unable to relax the knot in my chest. Very, very stressed. And inconsolable by Chris. My head feels full of blood, congested, a sign of soaring blood pressure I suspect.

I can't sleep. In the end I drift off, but only for a couple of hours at a time.

I had never heard of 'sleep obesity' until now, but Dr Eve Van Cauter has a doctorate in it. She conducted a series of studies showing that lack of sleep is associated with weight gain and she calls sleep deprivation 'the royal road to obesity'. At the hormonal level, lack of sleep affects cortisol levels which increases both glucose and insulin levels. In turn, this is likely to promote the development of insulin resistance, a risk factor for obesity and diabetes. Glucose tolerance tests showed that in order to maintain normal blood sugar, subjects, all of normal weight, needed to produce 30 per cent more insulin if they slept 6.5 hrs or less per night, compared with those who slept for seven hours or more.

In addition, the levels of leptin, the 'fullness hormone', were shown to be suppressed in those who were sleep deprived. They were therefore more likely to experience hunger when what they actually needed was sleep.

NEXT MORNING I re-read my draft reply to check that it is reasonable and pressed send. Within an hour, there's a call from our presenter.

'I looked at my email to you again this morning and I think it sounded really negative. I was tired, it was late, and I was trying to be crisp and get to the point. I will of course do whatever you think we need to do.'

OMG. A relief, to say the least.

If that had happened at midday, what would I have done? I suspect that a sudden urge for toast or biscuits or a croissant would have felt quite reasonable. Irresistible in fact.

Sobering fact #17: *When stressed, our body goes into survival mode: Cortisol, the 'stress hormone', is secreted, which can cause an increase in appetite.*

Harvard Health Publishing, 2011

CHAPTER 18

The burning of the bras

13st 5lb

Thursday, 5 July 2012

I sit with Bridget on the train. It's strange to see her away from Dartmoor. Her wild hair and wispy Celtic presence attracts a bit of attention, but we ignore it.

'I'm on a real odyssey today,' I tell her, 'from Devon to Bristol, on to London and then home.'

A quirk of her eyebrows tells me she knows all this. Of course she does, but it's hard to remember because she never speaks. Personally I feel the need to verbalise.

'You know it would all be much easier if you ever told me what's going on,' I put it to her mildly. There's no point in outright criticism. It might put her back up.

'OK, I accept that you're in charge.' She smirks a little, which is frankly disconcerting. 'But I am here too. I do my best to understand what you need, and how you're feeling, but sometimes it seems like a one-way trip. I mean that you never try to communicate with me – you just make me do stuff.'

I expect her to be impatient but she puts her hand over mine in a gesture of comfort. Then she astonishes me by taking my phone out of my hand – and tweeting me!

'Anything worth saying can be said in 140 characters or less,' she writes, tapping out the message with a sweep of the hand.

Well you can't expect me to agree with that. In my head I never shut up. Words tumble and flow through my brain like flotsam and jetsam, occasionally forming patterns which sometimes come out as speech, but often just drift around, forming and reforming. Her sage utterance is all very well, but it undermines everything I know about myself.

WHEN I WAS fifteen bra-burning was a phrase full of revolutionary fervour. It meant freedom from the shackles of man and marriage, and it heralded liberty and equality. Now it's a literal act – the destruction of seven old careworn bras that have seen finer days.

I text Chris, who has reached Chorley on day 6 of the cycle ride from hell (that's according to me – he's loving it). 'New bra 38E down from 42H!!! Tell no one or you'll never see either of them again.'

It's a brave act, to chuck out clothes of a previous size. This is the first cull I've had, although there are at least six pairs of trousers and jeans that won't stay up, even with belts, which I hope never to wear again.

Part of me wants to hang on to them. They are a security blanket, the answer to a barely articulated question, 'But what if I should slip ...? Have I really done with being seventeen stone?' Yes, I think I have, but I'm superstitious. If I chuck them, will it break this streak of luck that is enabling me to carry on?

Bridget has much to contribute on this, although as ever wordlessly. First of all, she hints that old and faded bras will not protect me from gaining weight. If I should ever gain again, the answer is to buy new bras of great technological wizardry to contain the puppies. OK, that's that bit dealt with.

Second – superstition. She growls at me. How dare I be superstitious? That suggests this whole process is about luck, but it's no such thing. Bridget is in charge and she's decided the time is right for a BMI of … I can't even bring myself to write it down. Sounds too certain and intentional. But not obese anyway.

Talking of which, I've just realised that I've moved out of the 'obese' and into the 'overweight' category for the first time in nearly twenty years. Currently on 29.9, down from 39.4. Not bad.

CHRIS RINGS TO chat every night at ten. Tonight he admits he thought I had properly lost it last week when I got that tricky email from the presenter. He was aware of me fretting all night, not sleeping, stressing. He was afraid he would have to abandon the trip, come home and spoon baby food into me until sanity returned. But I'm managing – the school run, two dog walks, work, a daily clothes wash, daily shop, nightly cook, washing up, writing, chatting to Orlando and then doing it all again. How do single parents cope?

In one sense what my literal bra-burning represents is totally contrary to feminism. Why did I feel I had to conform to a body stereotype, what pressures urged me to diet? But in another, it is liberation – from potential disease, from a condition amounting to a disability that I've lived with all my life. I'm throwing it off.

And yet on any given day if you asked me how it's going I would say it isn't – I feel stuck, unable to lose any more. Yes I've done well, but it's so slow now and I can't believe I can lose any more. It took me a month to lose the last pound for goodness sake.

What happens to Bridget if I succeed? Will she still be there even if we aren't talking about my weight? Well of course. Other issues in life need a careful inner eye. That's what I've come to think she is.

The great benefit of this exercise is that I'm learning to live at peace with her, at least on this one tricky issue of weight. Let's not presume beyond that.

13st 3lb

Saturday, 14 July 2012

CHRIS IS STILL away and things have settled down. We're obviously going to make it through. It's slow going. I limp onwards but my resolve is unshakable. Well, that's what people want to hear anyway. In fact, as you've probably gathered by now, that's not it at all. Unshakable ha ha ha. Shaken every day more like. But committed to patience and the long haul. It can't *not* work. Still.

I'm beginning to wonder whether I should lay quite so much power at Bridget's door. I feel disloyal saying so, having bent over backwards to revere her powers of decision, but is she really the final arbiter? I decide to write to Dr David Papineau, he of *In Our Time* fame, and ask him.

-----Original Message-----

From: Grace Kitto
To: Papineau, David
Subject: In Our Time

Dear David Papineau

You may remember that you appeared on In Our Time with Melvyn Bragg a couple of years ago, talking about developments in neuroscience. I was particularly struck by your description of Benjamin Libet's experiments, which seemed to indicate that decisions are made by the unconscious mind before the conscious mind is aware of them. You said that these experiments are now controversial, and they are presumably outdated – but you had brought them up, and referred to them as significant in the way we view the mind.

I have listened to that interview many times since, and have followed up by reading about Benjamin Libet, and about your own work. I've tried to find out if his experiments have been replicated since he first carried them out, using more modern methods and equipment. There seems to be a lot of conflicting material around. What I'm looking for is some sort of context – I would be most grateful if you could suggest some reading which would help me understand where this work on the brain is leading now.

Thinking, Fast and Slow by Daniel Kahneman seems to bear out Libet's hypothesis to some extent, don't you think? That's if you take Kahneman's system 1 to represent the unconscious ... But of course he is an economist who is delving into psychology, not a neurologist. I'd like to know where neurology is on this subject.

I hope this isn't a nuisance email! I have tried to find out what I can but feel I'm floundering, and would be very grateful for any help or pointers you can offer.

Kind regards

Grace

-----Original Message-----

From: Papineau, David
To: Grace Kitto

Dear Grace (if I may)

Sorry to be a bit slow replying. (And that wasn't a nuisance e-mail at all.)

Libet's work has been replicated, and there are lots of similar results around.

The standard response (or at least the one I think is sensible) to these results is that they show that the immediate control of our movements isn't in fact under conscious control, but pretty automatic (controlled by a 'system 1' if you like) – but that this doesn't show that conscious deliberation and intention-formation doesn't ever make a difference to what we do. But the kind of conscious deliberation that does matter is the kind of ('system 2') weighing up the pros and cons of different plans, and then committing yourself to one, which will then often involve complex series of actions, often in the quite distant future – quite different from sitting there waiting until you are moved to press the button, as in Libet's experiments.

I hope that makes sense. I have attached a recently finished PhD by a student of mine on just this topic, if you are interested in exploring further.

With best wishes

David

This is cheering evidence that Bridget is not the only Fat Controller in the village. It seems there is a sort of hierarchy of decision-making going on, in which we 'delegate' unimportant decisions to our unconscious, which is also busy looking out for danger and making sense of our surroundings.

But when we have a significant dilemma, the power of rational thought comes into its own. With system 2 we weigh things up, learn from the past, plan ahead and work out how to make changes (none of which system 1 is good at).

There's some rebalancing of power going on here. I'm subject to Bridget's whims, but not as much as I thought at the beginning. That doesn't mean my first approach to her was wrong. I had to go through the process of learning to make peace with her and to respect her before I could make any headway – when it comes to addictive behaviour, system 1 decision-making is key. But it's good to know that she's not in sole charge and that I do indeed have the power to change my mind.

I wonder if I should talk to her about this. Could be a bit awkward. I'm not sure how she'd take it.

BRIDGET IS STALKING around her cave, refusing to look at me. I try to reason with her but can't get anywhere. Because she doesn't speak, I'm not quite sure what the matter is. Now is obviously not the moment to raise the idea that she's not all-powerful over my decisions.

She paces to and fro, distracted and muttering. Then it dawns on me. Today a pretty, lively girl called Selina came into the office. She was amazed at how much weight I've lost, gushed and cooed.

'You've done so well. It's amazing. You must have such will-power! I really don't think I could do what you've done.'

I try to be gracious and accept the compliment, but it doesn't feel exactly like willpower to me, but a sort of painful protracted compromise, a continual wrangling. Like when they say after peace talks that they've 'hammered out an agreement' and it sounds like an inbuilt contradiction, the violence of the image fighting with the so-called peace. I've got internal peace talks going on all day. I'm trying to accommodate Bridget and, to be fair, although in some ways she appears completely uncompromising, she's accommodating me too. She's letting me do it.

But it seems Bridget resents the very idea of 'willpower'. It annoys her. It sounds to her as though I'm claiming victory when in fact she holds all the cards. But I wasn't. I was equally uncomfortable being given all the credit. I know I have to tread carefully, be tactful and not presume.

Who knew she could be so touchy?

Sobering fact #18: *Having previously been on a diet has been determined as a predictor of weight gain.*

Frontiers in Psychology, 2013

CHAPTER 19

In which I do not adjust my seat belt

13st 5lb

Saturday, 11 August 2012

'Bridget – are you there?'

Silly question. She's always there. 'I'm a bit confused. I get the feeling that you don't like change much.'

She's splitting bamboo stakes for some purpose I can't work out, tying them together and storing them. I wonder idly if she gardens.

'So – if that's right … why are you sanctioning this? My visits – letting me move on?'

She hands me a bunch of the bamboos. I watch her and then copy. It's surprisingly easy to find a purchase point, and then split each stem vertically down its length. Soon, I'm doing it faster than Bridget. When I've finished the lot, I tie them into a neat bundle and pass them back. There's a flicker of acknowledgement.

'So you like help then.'

But she has her back to me, and is stacking up the piles of bamboo inside the mouth of her cave. It seems to be some kind of store cupboard.

'Will you be here tomorrow?' A level look reminds me – she is of course always here.

'I'll come back then. There's something I'd like to bring you.'

I turn away, hoping to intrigue her. But she's off across the hillside. I've already lost her attention.

CHRIS CAME HOME a few days ago. He stood in the kitchen chatting to us both about his trip and I could see straight away that during his three weeks away, Orlando has outstripped him in height. At not quite fifteen it's remarkable, particularly as Chris is six foot four. Only a few millimetres but it's a distinct gap. Orlando's very pleased with himself.

'Move over, Shorty – I want to look in the mirror'.

How our pasts comes back to bite us. Chris has called Orlando 'Shorty' all his life. Now the tables have well and truly turned.

'You cheeky little scrote.'

'Not so little ...'

It's obvious that Chris is proud and nettled in equal measure.

WE'VE BEEN AWAY for a short beach holiday. I'm in the middle of a hefty filming schedule and a week was all the time we could spare.

I have eaten very well – masses of fruit, very little bread and only one pudding the whole time we were away. I am hopeful that all is well. No loss, no gain, would be ideal.

In the plane on the way over I was delighted to find that I could clip on my seat belt without adjusting it first. Only those of us who have been seriously obese know how excruciating it feels to extend the belt to its max, and then breathe in, desperate to shut it without attracting attention. But this time a full seven or eight inches of unused strap lay in my lap.

Our holiday in the sun was very leisurely. Orlando water skied. He's found his balance, so only had to stop when his hands hurt. Chris struggled to keep upright but finally managed a whole seventeen seconds, caught on deathless video. I tried, but kept falling over. My greatest achievement was that I put on a life jacket and fastened it without a second thought. They used to be called Mae Wests, not so funny

157

if your boobs are too big to squeeze into them. We drifted through the days and came back brown and relaxed.

Driving home from the airport, we stopped at a service station and I queued to buy coffees. Virgin had supplied us with a very odd breakfast on the plane: omelette, bacon and sausages but not a bit of toast, croissant or brioche to be seen. If there's one time of day that I think carbs are essential, it's breakfast.

By mid-morning my stomach was rumbling. Standing in line at Starbucks I looked around for what I could eat. There were massive breakfast muffins, dense calorie-laden nuggets of sugar in the form of strawberry or caramel shortcake, or side-plate sized monster cookies (at a mere 470 calories a go).

My eye had just settled on a plain croissant which, although butter-laden, was probably the safest option, when I became aware of the woman in front of me. She was about thirty-five, dressed in black jeans and a black t-shirt, her hair tied back in a girlish ponytail. She stood well. She had attitude. And she was at least twenty stone. She had the manner of someone who isn't letting her weight get in her way – quite cool, defiant even.

Her order came – a frosted cupcake the size of a football and a grande hot chocolate topped with whipped cream and a marshmallow twizzle. I identified with her so much that I badly wanted to lean across and say something to her – but what? Anything I could think of would be crass and judgemental, however kindly meant.

I could see Chris and Orlando looking at me, dreading that I would speak to her. Neither of them would do that in a trillion years, but they both know I'm capable of it. I suppose that seeing her choices (which would once have been mine) made me wish I could speak to my past self. I would have pointed out that it takes hundreds of small decisions to eat a snack like that – not even a meal, mind you – to put on each stone. Then even more similar decisions in the opposite direction to take it off again.

That's why losing weight requires such patience. Immediately

I turned on my heel, marched down the corridor to the super-market and bought some fruit – a tub of pineapple and mango slices, and a banana. And silently thanked Bridget that I could.

You might read this and think how dare I make assumptions about that woman, and jump to the conclusion that she would prefer to lose weight. I'm not saying she wants to, but the point is that there is a very convincing reason why she should – she's more likely to die younger than she should as a result of eating that way. And yes, I know this sounds like Chris talking to me down through the years before Cadover Bridge.

I'm quite hungry now. Would like to go into the kitchen, make myself some toast and slather it with peanut butter. But will not. That's not to say never again; on some unspecified day I will consider, be mindful – and then decide that it's appropri-ate and proportionate to eat peanut butter on toast. I will do it and enjoy it. But not on a whim, without thinking it through. Or worst of all, finding myself standing in the kitchen, half eaten toast and peanut butter in hand, looking at what's left and wondering how it got there, having munched without tasting.

I cannot be the only person this happens to. It's a terrible trick of the mind that catapults us into narcotic overeating. Habit, self-sabotage, lack of self-worth or defensive weight gain – let's just stop it right now.

I began this enterprise resenting the fact that every book and magazine about dieting is full of menus and dishes, adverts for food and articles about food. Too much food, in fact. I try not to dwell on it here. I'm writing about how the issues around obesity affect me, not the thing itself. But every now and then we must name the demon, and shame him back into his box.

ALONGSIDE MY MOTHER, with her wonderful cooking and lavish overeating, there was my stepmother. She inherited us, the four youngest of my mother's six kids, and eventually had five of her own too, but it wasn't clear why. 'I should never have had children,' she would say. She didn't mention stepchildren.

She wasn't a foodie. I piece these things together slowly, like a detective. So my loving, flamboyant, but largely absent mother prepared delicious, exotic dishes in abundance – and overate. My less kindly stepmother showed little interest in food except that she was controlling about it. They both delegated too much responsibility for cooking to me, too young. They both 'punished' me, as it seemed to me, for overeating. Go figure.

There is a particular frozen moment, remembered with pain by my brothers, my sister and me. It was Crispin's twelfth birthday and he had just started at secondary school. He had about a dozen friends to afternoon tea and there was a big beautiful cake which all of us little ones were invited to come and queue up for. When it was my turn, my stepmother stopped proceedings, and in front of all these unknown teenagers, pointed at me and said, 'Are you sure you should have any? Do you really think you should?'

Her meaning was unmistakable. I was too fat to be allowed cake. Not too fat to be summoned to queue for it though. My eyes filled and I didn't know where to put myself. I salivated, not for cake, but in fear and shame. Crispin and Belinda bundled me out, stuffing cake into my hand. I shiver at the memory of that moment.

On another occasion, still in Cornwall, all of us kids were milling round in the kitchen when my father suddenly appeared. He was a big, muscular man, six feet tall, but he moved exceptionally quietly and it was often with shock that we would register his silent presence. He was grinning, holding up a banana skin.

In his deep velvet voice: 'Who's been eating fruit in the bog?'

He said he'd found a pile of rotten apple cores, orange peel and banana skins posted out of the window of the lav on the landing. They were stacking up round the base of the japonica in the flower bed behind the loo.

It was me, of course. I did it. I must have been hungry and scared. My dad was amused, but my stepmother was not.

He wandered off. 'For god's sake, chuck them in the bin next time.'

There wouldn't be a next time. He had no idea how much trouble I was in. He wouldn't have made it so public if he had. There's that ping, like an elastic band, another pinprick of pain. But let me be clear. I am recalling this for the purposes of my current detective work. Blaming your parents, and indeed step-parents, is fruitless by the time you reach my age. It's not blame allocation that interests me. Despite all this delving into the past, the answers to my predicament lie right here, in the present.

I'm interrogating the past because I want to understand my own conditioning and challenge it. I'm challenging it right now.

A COUPLE OF days ago, I was on the train, on my way to London, when a very drunk man in my compartment complained about me talking too loud and too long on the phone.

He lurched across to my table and said grandly, 'Really not on. Not. Mobile phones are the scourge of the age. Meantersay. End of civilised conversation as we know it.'

It so happened that there was a bit of a drama going on at work. We had a shoot where one thing after another was going wrong and two presenters were up in arms. They had fallen out, were barely speaking, and wouldn't travel in the same car or eat together. They each thought the other was behaving very badly. They could just about put on a show of good relations during filming but it was a very precarious situation. How do you get a good atmosphere on screen if you're raging off screen? My sympathies were pretty evenly divided, despite a passing urge to bang their heads together. I also wanted to support the poor crew, who were stuck in the middle.

I was contrite to my travelling companion. There are few things more irritating than being forced to listen to someone else's conversation when you were expecting the peace and quiet of a long train journey. I apologised profusely and hurried out into the howling corridor to finish my calls.

When I returned to my seat, he staggered over to my table and plonked himself down. He took out a business card and slapped it down in front of me.

'I'm Shtuart. An inshnational economicsh expert for the BBC.' This with a flourish, as if I wouldn't believe him, the card as proof. I said how sorry I was to have disturbed him, and explained briefly what was going on.

'Wait a minute. They're presenters, right? Not your problem. Both adultsh. Both paid to do a job. End of.'

How different is the world inside our great institutions. In a small production company we can't afford to take that sort of bullish line. It's vital to us that everyone gets on and plays nice.

'S'Ridiculous. Not your problem ...'

He was gearing up to rant, I could see, but at that moment my mobile went off again. He turned sharply away, offended at the interruption, and I ran back out into the corridor to take my call. When I got back he was still at my table, radiating drunken disapproval. He had clearly forgotten that he hadn't been invited to join me in the first place. I wanted to laugh, but he turned out to be good company and we talked all the way to London – with a lot more of the same sort of advice thrown in. It was refreshing to listen to his bracing analysis of my situation, but I was never going to act on it.

When Chris heard about this encounter he immediately assumed that Stuart was coming on to me. That it actually hadn't crossed my mind shows how long it's been since that happened. Good lord.

Sobering fact #19: *An estimated 7.1 per cent of deaths (35,820) are attributable to elevated BMI in England and Wales in 2014. Each individual lost twelve years on average.*

Institute of Economic Affairs, 2017

CHAPTER 20

Are we nearly there yet?

13st 2lb

Saturday, 25 August 2012

NO, WE ARE not is the rough but truthful answer. We are not nearly there. We may be two thirds of the way down this long and winding road but it winds on right out of sight. No surprise to find nothing shifting despite another week's strenuous efforts.

﹀

I'm on the tor, sweet wood smoke wafting my way as I head towards the fire.

'Hi.' I stumble over. 'How are you?'

There's a faraway look in Bridget's eyes. She barely acknowledges me.

'Why am I so filled with doubt about this process?'

I see a quirk of her eyebrow. 'Words, words, words,' she seems to be saying. 'Why all these words? Why can't you just get on with it and stop everlasting talking about everything?!'

'Oh good,' I say. 'Then it's OK?'

She nods and settles back to look at the fire once more.

'Would you like me to go?' A little sideways shake of the head. She doesn't mind. She is contemplative and doesn't have a lot of time for me, but is OK with my presence, neither welcoming nor unwelcoming. This is strangely comforting.

'So the doubting backdrop is just noise. I can ignore it. In fact

I must ignore it – don't give it oxygen. Don't pay it any attention. Just keep doing what I'm doing?'

She pokes the fire, which sparks into life, flames leaping up to illuminate her face.

I think I understand. I haven't really wavered, and even though the doubts don't go, they haven't changed what I've been doing. It doesn't matter that fears and worries break through. As long as I keep a straight path, doubts won't make any difference.

———

PART OF BEING human is to live with a burble of voices in your head – all your own – agreeing and disagreeing with every thought you formulate and every sentence you utter. Thinking wildly contradictory things all at the same time – it's not working, it's too hard, I want Liquorice Allsorts.

But also flickers of encouragement, I've come a long way, it's easy, I like where I am now, I can have Liquorice Allsorts later.

A series of constant checks and balances, feeling your way across the quicksand. It's the noise in our heads. It's there to learn from, there to help us work things out, not to be taken literally.

AS EVER, I'M battling with the physical challenge as well as the psychological one, that is, what should I actually be eating? The answer is much less obvious than all the diet books and magazines make out – and they don't agree anyway.

My daily menu at the moment looks something like this:

- Breakfast is always fruit plus wholemeal toast, either a poached egg or one piece of bacon, no butter, and sometimes one teaspoonful of marmalade or jam (200–250 calories in all).
- Lunch is soup (120–160 calories depending on what sort).
- Lots of fruit during the day (300–400 calories).

- Dinner is usually pasta, meat and veg or occasionally risotto, though rarely, because it's surprising how little rice you get in a modest portion (400–500 calories).

It's worth recording for two reasons. First, to demonstrate that my calories intake is low, at around 1200 calories per day including fruit. Second, to show that it's far from starvation rations. It's balanced and moderate. If there was any justice, it would do the trick. But there is no justice.

This is where I miss having an intelligent support group. Most people I share this problem with are quick to judge. Either they assume that I'm kidding myself and I'm actually eating more than I say, or they worry that I'm on some ridiculously low calorie self-punishment regime.

Neither is the case. I'm eating moderately, but obviously not moderately enough to keep losing. I begin to suspect that less is known about weight loss than we can possibly credit given the vast array of books, articles, websites and products, never mind the so-called experts who declare for one diet or another.

There are copious articles on the web on 'How to Break Through a Plateau'. They all start with a hearty call to hang on in there (doing that) and recheck your calorie intake (on it).

They refer to BMR (basal metabolic rate), which is the number of calories used to breathe, keep your heart pumping, your body temperature stable and to replace cells. In other words, what you use simply to stay alive.

The bad news is that your BMR drops once you lose weight. In other words, the less you weigh, the less food you need to keep your body functioning. So as a diet progresses your calorie intake needs to drop too if you want to keep losing.

The formula for working out BMR is based on age, height, weight and activity level and the easiest way to check it is via an online calculator, although it needs lab conditions to be completely accurate. My BMR, based on one such online approximation, gives me a resting rate of 1435 calories (if I stay in bed all day). With moderate activity it tells me I can consume 1730 calories without gaining weight.

It is widely quoted that to lose one pound 'costs' 3000–3500 calories. In other words, you need to consume 3000 calories fewer than you burn for each pound you want to lose. So in theory, if I eat 1200 calories per day for a week, and keep up moderate activity, I will have 'saved' about 450 calories per day, so 3150 per week, and will comfortably lose a pound at the end of that week.

The only problem is that I've been putting this theory to the test, and it hasn't been working.

NEVERTHELESS, AFTER EIGHT weeks with barely any movement, I've finally cracked four stone. It's much slower than anyone tells you it will be. The voice in my head kept telling me that it was never going to happen, and that I was stuck for good and all. But at the same time feedback has been continually positive, so I assume that inches have been coming off, if not pounds. I can feel it too, like the tide gradually going out, even if the scales haven't agreed.

To give myself a fighting chance I've given up soup for lunch and have an apple or an orange instead. At the beginning, if you remember, I fretted at the thought of soup without a roll for lunch. A year and a half on, lunch itself has become a cursory snack and I don't miss it.

Changing my attitude to the speed of this thing is the key. As long as I'm losing, I'll try to be content. That's not to say there isn't a constant nagging voice in my head complaining about how slow it is. Like a hypercritical ancient relative, never shutting up, always right, never giving in, my inner critic just loves to tell me where I'm going wrong. But you and I know that I'm actually going fairly right.

Chris finds it strange, after so many years together, to have to get to know this new me, an unfamiliar size and shape. 'There are lovely bones and muscles coming through,' he says.

BLACK TEA WITH toast and jam for breakfast. Brown toast, no butter, one teaspoon of homemade apricot jam I bought at a farm nearby. Delicious. It took me back nearly forty years to my days as an au pair in Italy for an Italian-American family. Two children of five and three were in my charge, and while their parents were in Greece on a sailing holiday, the kids and I went to stay with their Italian grandmother, known as La Nonna.

She didn't speak English and I was slowly learning Italian so we communicated in French (shaky AS level on my part but I was game to give it a go). At the same time I pored over an Italian grammar every night and got hopelessly confused between the two languages. I drove myself nuts saying 'si' when I meant 'oui', let alone whole sentences.

Every morning I had breakfast in the kitchen, a bowl full of caffè macchiato the size of a bucket and piles of fresh, crusty white bread with a springy fragrant inside. I ate it slathered with almost white butter and home made apricot jam, softly crunchy from the kernels left in it. It must have contained about ten times the number of calories as today's version. Delicious but deadly – an early staging post on my disastrous career in calories.

There were three family members living in this huge house, surrounded by a walled garden and electric gates, and supported by a clutch of maids. They were La Nonna, La Zia (great-aunt to the children) and Zio Bruno, son of La Nonna, who was in his early forties, hopeless, hugely fat, permanently unhappy and prone to enormous scenes. He had a sort of batman known as Il Cacciatore (the huntsman) who came to attend him every day. There was a pretence that they would go out shooting together, but the main job of Il Cacciatore seemed to be to keep Bruno content.

'Stai calmo, Bruno, calmo ...' he would murmur, keeping at bay Bruno's fearsome agitation.

But every few days there would be a sudden explosion, huge cries of, '*Mamma, Zia, Mamma, Zia, venite subito,*' and a rush of footsteps as these two gentle old ladies hurried to his side. Once they reached his ground floor apartment, they were screamed at and cried at, howls of rage and frustration filling the house. La Nonna and La Zia muttered comfort and commiseration, love and compassion, and eventually Bruno's drama would subside, his rage turning to loud sobbing.

I thought he had a pretty cushy number. La Nonna was embarrassed, but stoic. After every one of these scenes she and I would meet over the dining table and converse in a mixture of French (mine hesitant, hers fluent) and Italian. She wanted to excuse Bruno.

'*Bruno è sensibile,*' she said. Yeah I bet he is, I thought uncharitably – sensitive to his own feelings, rather than to his mother's or his aunt's.

La Nonna fed me the first Parma ham I had ever tasted. I was shocked when she told me it was '*crudo*' – raw – and I could barely eat it, not understanding that though it was uncooked, it was cured. We sat in the formal dining room together, dark wood everywhere, stray shafts of sunlight catching the crystal glasses lined up on her dark wood dresser, dust turning in the haze as we made conversation in faltering French.

La Nonna always dressed in layers of black, grey and navy blue, her white hair elegantly folded into a bun at the back of her neck. Beautiful and gracious, and very kind. I tried my hardest to disguise my disgust and eat the ham, but at nineteen it wasn't a very subtle try. The next time melon and Parma ham was served for dinner, mine came unadorned.

'I could see that you didn't like it,' she said.

I was mortified but grateful. I wish I had understood then that melon and Parma ham was a perfect food for me. Not a carb in sight – unlike the delicious bread and apricot jam.

This morning I sit here enjoying just a taste of apricot jam again. Taken judiciously, as part of a plan, with no damage done.

LOOKING THIS THING straight in the face. I've lost twelve
pounds over twenty-four weeks. That means a steady half
pound a week over the last six months. I'm struggling to adopt
an appropriate attitude to that.

On one hand, it's a shockingly meagre loss considering the
effort I feel I've put in. WW still says I should be losing 1–2
pounds per week. I know lots of people who can lose that much
for a week or two, almost no one who can keep it up long term.
At this rate it'll take another year to lose the final two stone to
get to a BMI of 25.

On the other hand, I'm still not exercising much – too busy,
too bored – but even so I've managed to lose. Who cares how
long it takes? And where's the deadline?

I veer between these two points of view. More often the
negative one sticks and there is a constant white noise in my
head which I have to make efforts to ignore, 'You've done
OK but it's over now, doesn't matter how hard you try, it isn't
shifting ...'

13st 2lb

Wednesday, 12 September 2012

JUST TO CHECK that I'm not missing anything by not attending,
I decide to drop in on a WW class. Nothing has changed except
the soft sell of WW products from the class leader has become
a bit harder. She gives a talk 'How to avoid making bad choices
in a coffee shop', which is packed with shocking stats on the
calories in a skinny latte. Peppered throughout are reminders of
the low calorie hot chocolate sachets on sale at the back of the
room, as well as numerous other snacks.

'Caramel bars and chocolate shortbread are on special offer
today ladies!'

These diets products are laid out on a long table along one wall of the hall. I find myself spending over £23 on a load of things I don't need, including sachets of bolognaise sauce, chiding myself as I do so ('You idiot – you can make that!'), chewing gum, fruit-flavoured sweets (a whole packet is only one point) and, yes, caramel bars. I'm such a sucker.

The diet industry is not our friend. This is clear to me, seeing all these goods on display. Just as diet magazines are full of adverts for food, articles on food and photographs of food, it feeds the compulsive streak in us all. And we keep on going back. In fact, I'm the ideal client, good enough at a programme like this one to lose a lot and testify to its success, but never free of it, never let back into the community to go it alone, always here, paying my subs.

Afterwards I stay behind to talk to the class leader to see if she can offer any insight; even more, to see if I can bear the idea of coming regularly. I tell her what I've achieved so far using WW online and how slowly I'm losing now. I ask if there's anything she can suggest that will help.

She gives a sweet smile. 'You can't have a big enough calorie deficit, that's the thing. If you did, you'd still be losing.'

'What a cow.' The thought arises before I can censor it. There must be truth in what she says, logically speaking. But the thing is, I'm sticking to the WW plan, and it's just not working. So, how dare she?

Right then. Austerity measures.

'Why don't you ask Bridget why you've stalled?' Chris drops her name into the conversation as though she's an old friend who I might go and natter to about anything. Are we both crazy? You decide.

I have a feeling that she'll have little to offer on the subject, but I might as well give it a go.

'Bridget – why is it so slow?'

She shrugs. I really don't think she knows.

'Is there anything you could do to help?'

Pursed lips. Discreet smile.

'You could make it a little simpler for me to do what I've decided to do. Make me less conflicted.'

A small shake of the head and she turns away.

She could make it easier, but I'm assuming she won't.

'DROP THE APRICOT jam,' I think I can hear you say. Alright, but as well as losing weight I want to enjoy life and that means enjoying food too, all the more delicious for being a rare, sparing treat.

Sobering fact #20: *80 per cent French women are thought to be on a diet at any given time.*

Gabrielle Deydier, *On ne naît pas grosse*, 2017
Observer, 2017

CHAPTER 21

Brain food

13st 1lb

Saturday, 22 September 2012

ONE OF DANIEL Kahneman's experiments left me with a question. It's that one where he set subjects the task of memorising a series of digits. Meanwhile, they were offered a choice of two desserts, chocolate cake or fruit salad. He says, if you remember, that if we are thinking hard with 'system 2', the effort depletes our glucose levels and 'system 1' is drawn to sweet snacks to keep up its momentum. What this left me wondering is whether we burn more calories when we think hard because this prompts us to eat more, and whether anyone has measured this increase.

Adult human brains apparently weigh between 2.6 and 3 pounds, about 2 per cent of the average person's weight. Brain activity consumes a disproportionate amount of energy at 20 per cent of our BMR (basal metabolic rate – see previous chapter), which equates to around 260 calories per day. So even a large percentage shift on that number would make only a modest difference to overall consumption.

In one (admittedly tiny) study, fourteen Canadian women were allocated one of three activities. One set were asked to summarise a paragraph, another to complete computerised memory tasks and the third set just sat around. Afterwards, they helped themselves to a buffet lunch. Those whose brains had been busy ate on average 200 calories more than those who had not. Their blood sugar levels fluctuated but not in a consistent way and their heart rates, blood pressure, cortisol levels and self-reported anxiety were all higher. The article in *Scientific American*, 'Does Thinking Really Hard Burn More Calories?', hypothesised that they were 'stress eating'.

It's interesting that they ate more, even by a small amount. But what does 'stress eating' actually mean in this context? Does it mean their cortisol levels (the 'stress hormone') were particularly high? No, cortisol was only part of the picture.

I love the way these phrases are bandied about. They were alert and responsive as a result of the challenges, it is true. Personally, I'd like to find out more before applying this kind of catch-all phrase to their behaviour. In my view, it's just not specific enough to be helpful.

I've brought Bridget a slice of chocolate cake (not my favourite). I want to see what she does with it. It's another kind of test.

There's a tree stump which doubles as a table near to her cave. I make a tidy little picnic for her – a side plate with the cake on it, a fork and a paper napkin.

Just as it's ready, she appears. She looks at it and gives a curt nod of thanks, but makes no move towards it.

I sit down and warm my hands at the fire. Bridget trots to and fro, busying herself with her cooking pots. She walks round the cake.

'Are you going to eat it?' I really want to know.

She puts her head on one side, and makes a face. 'Maybe,' she seems to say. She seems completely unfazed by having it there. She might eat it or she might not.

'I'm not sure I understand. Aren't you tempted?'

A quick shake of the head – no, not tempted.

'Is it just me then? Am I on the rack and you're free to take it or leave it?'

She comes as near to laughing as I've ever seen.

'What drama!' she implies.

Now I'm really confused. Would it be different if I'd brought her something I prefer, like carrot cake or a flapjack? Would she prefer that too?

I suspect not. She's just not as anxiously caught up with food as me. How odd. How intriguing.

She barely looks up as I go.

I'll tell you one thing. She's a lot more self-possessed than I am.

⁓

THE WW PROGRAMME has helped me lose weight for eighteen months and given me a fantastic start. But now it's stopped working, I don't feel loyal to it. Dieters sometimes get a semi-religious zeal about their particular regime which I find hard to understand. It's not the plan that's got me where I am. It's me and Bridget, working in harmony. If I need a new diet, so be it.

Weight Watchers has been a great ally though. In the right circumstances I would do it again. What I'll take with me from it is the discipline of smaller portions, its flexibility, because almost any food can be factored into the diet, and its balanced approach. What I can't quite bring myself to do is to cancel my membership.

Chris thinks this is loony and I can only defend it by saying that I want to keep my online weight tracker going. But really it's superstition – this is how I got where I am now and I can't quite bear to bin it yet.

My next strategy is to road test a series of diets to see how they work for me. The 5:2 diet has had a good press and it appeals. The basic idea is that if you fast on two days and eat normally on five, you will lose weight. I've decided to try it.

Word on the street is that many of the staff from our local hospital are also giving the 5:2 diet a go. Our friend Tim, a consultant, explains that he likes the idea of resting the pancreas once or twice a week. He thinks it just might be, as claimed, some protection against diabetes. As that's one of my principle objectives, it's reassuring and makes me think it's a great regime for me.

13st 1lb

Tuesday, 25 September 2012

THE FASTING DAYS on the 5:2 diet don't involve zero consumption, just heavily restricted intake at 500–600 calories per day. Today was the first day, extra tough because I was travelling, which is always challenging. The only food available on trains is carb heavy, loaded with fat and sugar. One day someone will invent a food brand which is nutrient-rich, tasty and satisfying. Not today unfortunately. But even so, the day went well.

Friday, 28 September 2012

I'VE EATEN NORMALLY for the rest of the week (that is, a kind of relaxed WW-diet normal) until today, Friday, my second 'fasting' day. I got home tonight so ravenously hungry that I couldn't resist eating – a lot. Vegetable curry, sag aloo, rice and naan. I didn't weigh any of this but am morally certain it was off the scale. Then I followed it up with not one but twelve squares of chocolate and a pot of low calorie rice pudding (low calorie?! Yes. What can I say?).

Well indeed. Scotched before I've really begun.

⁓

Somewhere in the space between cooking and eating, I spared a thought for Bridget. I didn't visit her, probably because I didn't want to hear what she would have to say. I phoned her.

When she picked up I started to babble, 'Look, I don't really know why I'm calling because I don't think there's anything you can say that will stop me. I really am so hungry that I can't stop myself. For the first time in ages I am just going to eat what I like. I'll take the consequences and get back on the wagon tomorrow, but tonight I just have to eat. Just thought I'd let you know.'

I put the phone down – and only then realised that I hadn't given her a moment to respond. She doesn't speak anyway so it can't have made much difference. All I can say is that it was good to make contact. It might not have actually changed what I did, but it was a nod at some kind of self-control.

13st 1lb

Saturday, 29 September 2012

I HAD ASSUMED that my unstoppable hunger was the result of the fast day, but this morning all became clear. I woke with a banging headache and a slight temperature. I spent the day feeling odd and out of sorts, unsmiling and uncomfortable, obviously with some kind of virus.

Bad eating continued. Lots of grazing, too many carbs, uncounted excess. Of course fears that I've lost my way begin to stalk me. Will I look back and think this is the day that I blew it? How do I get back on track? And so on.

Sunday, 30 September 2012

BUT BY THE end of the second groggy day I started to feel well again and so this morning (Sunday) I am back on plan 5:2, a huge relief. Panic subsides.

12st 13lb

Saturday, 6 October 2012

SO – INTO THE twelve stones. This is extraordinary. I'm on the normal spectrum for the first time in many years, elated, but

I've had to be rigorous to achieve it, and am not counting my chickens.

A stone and three quarters to go. It feels like a distant oasis – a place of rest and nourishment, shining in a desert of dieting. This, by the way, is a Bad Thought because it suggests that a diet is a hard slog, and a journey, and that there'll be an end to it eventually. Not the way to look at it.

These are permanent lifestyle changes. Meanwhile, I still spend a lot of time just a bit hungry, which is appropriate because I am losing weight. At some point I'll have to learn to eat like a normal person, neither losing nor gaining. That'll be odd.

I've passed another milestone without even noticing: getting back into my wedding dress. I put it on now and prance round the garden in it like a child dressing up in her mum's high heels. It's a bit loose actually.

A FLASHBACK THIS morning to a camping trip a few years ago, when Orlando was small. We went with another family, close friends of ours. Their son, Jack, is a year older than Orlando, and at the time he was going through one of those phases when children know best about absolutely everything. He knew the best way to the south of France, the best way to cook a sausage and only way to put up a tent. It was, to say the least, annoying. But we love our friends and trusted that he would grow out of it (he did) and so hung on in there.

But one night we were driving back to our campsite in the hot French twilight, after a long baking day of sightseeing, when Jack began to taunt Orlando. About me.

'Your mum is really fat,' he said. Dead silence in the car – each one of the four adults present was, I imagine, silently willing themselves anywhere else but here, now, in this car. Orlando squirmed.

'Why is your mum so fat?'

'She's not really fat.' Orlando struck out, loyal and desperate.

'She is though. She's really, really fat.'

'She's lovely and she's not.' Orlando's eyes were pricking – he obviously wanted to cry. Me too. Utter humiliation; even worse, totally undefendable. How can you answer back to a six-year-old? I smiled and kissed the top of Orlando's head, no clue what to say to make it easier for everyone. Our friends were totally silenced too, I'm sure out of deep embarrassment.

Seeing Orlando's distress Jack piped up, 'Oh I get it, she's really fat but you love her anyway!' As though it was a revelation.

'Yes I do,' said Orlando, nestling close to me. I wanted to laugh out loud, gratitude to my boy and public shame going hand in hand. I felt like a pathetic fool for minding so much.

Painful and humiliating though this incident was, once out of that car Chris and I had a laugh over it. For me, the kind of laugh that makes your mouth twist.

That night in camp I heard a murmur of voices in the tent next to us. I couldn't hear the words, but the soft relentless voice of my dear friend Mandy, Jack's mum, talking, talking, talking, suddenly gave way to a roar of distress. I think she must have been explaining to him very gently where he had gone wrong.

Sobering fact #21: *'Obesity is the new smoking, and it represents a slow-motion car crash in terms of avoidable illness and rising health care cost.'*

Simon Stevens, CEO NHS England, 2014

CHAPTER 22

Neck or nothing

12st 8lb

Saturday, 16 February 2013

We've come to visit Stonehenge. We stay in a chintzy bed and breakfast nearby. Lying open-eyed in the darkness, I drop in to visit Bridget.

It's the first time I've seen where she sleeps. I had imagined her cold and lonely at night on her barren hill top, but no, the depths of her cave are cosy, with woven wall hangings in red and orange wool, a bright patchwork quilt and a soft duvet.

Bridget is about to go to bed herself. I feel privileged to be allowed in to her private sanctuary, but as she's quite happy, and so am I, we have little to say to each other. I soon drop off.

<hr />

I DON'T KNOW how I named her Bridget. She came to me, fully formed and ready for action, like Athena, who sprang fully armed from the head of her father Zeus after a blow to his skull from Hephaestus, blacksmith to the gods. Zeus had had a headache and asked Hephaestus to smite him on the bonce to cure it. Hephaestus smote away and the result was Athena, goddess of wisdom, courage and inspiration among many other things, strategy, maths and warfare included. She was a goddess of many parts.

Brigid is a Celtic name and a Celtic goddess, and she has parallels with Athena. Healing, wisdom and fire all belong to her. She was the bringer of fertility and the one who inspired poets and blacksmiths.

In this prehistoric landscape it feels right to think of my Bridget. In my imagination, she has an archaic quality, a sense of holding deeper knowledge than I have access to in my waking self. Perhaps she is a way of recognising the essence of what I feel, undiluted by pressures, influences and received ideas.

My mother was Scottish and my father Cornish. They both identified as Celtic, but jokily. 'Bloody Sassenachs,' my mother would mutter, as a fond term of abuse. Never serious, but uttered nevertheless.

ON THE WAY back to Devon, we drop in see my sister Julia and take her out to lunch.

'You watch,' I say to Chris and Orlando. 'I bet she still doesn't say anything about my weight.'

'But you've lost five stone – she must!'

Sure enough, no mention. We eat at a local pub and when it comes to pudding, I decline.

'Very virtuous,' she says.

That's the closest it comes.

Well, maybe I just have to accept that this is my obsession, not everyone else's too.

THE 5:2 DIET seems to be doing the trick and the reward is a good weigh-in. Not quite the best, but then there was that frenzied day last week. How could I have been so self-destructive? It's taken me a whole week to undo the damage. At least I've learned to do that straight away.

Chris sends me roses at work on my birthday, for only the second time in twenty-three years. Orlando offers to cook supper, which touches me very much.

'Lovely. What will you make?'

'Anything you like,' he is insouciant, full of confidence, 'as long as it doesn't have meat in it.' I go for risotto and he suggests butternut squash and sage. It's delicious.

I've been editing for the last few days, a tension-inducing job with late nights and sweaty palms. Unexpectedly I bump into an editor on another project in the kitchen and he pats me on the shoulder.

'I must say you're looking very good these days.' It feels like an extra birthday present.

I REDISCOVERED MY neck this week. My grandmother used to say I didn't have one, but then she was a 1930s diva with a neck like a swan.

There's been a double or even triple chin for years, hiding the place where a neck should be.

I'm an archaeologist and I've been on a dig, looking for the remains of a neck and finally found it. Now it's back, it's no big deal. Of course I have a neck, don't you? It's so easy to forget what we've achieved and remember only our deficits. Note to self – this is an achievement.

'DON'T YOU GO too far now.' Anna is severe. We've worked together for so long that she takes the inside track and feels she can lay down the law with me.

'They say that over forty you have to choose between your face and your arse. Don't choose your arse.'

I giggle but am secretly exultant. Right on cue. I've been waiting for this moment and am enjoying it enormously. For the first time ever someone thinks it's possible I'm getting too thin. At well over twelve stone! Hilarious.

As a matter of fact I wouldn't trust my own instincts about what I should weigh for one minute and that's why I'm aiming at around BMI 25. It's an objective goal and can't be distorted by my skewed sense of size.

It's not just Anna. The latest small drop appears to be

awakening anxieties among several of my friends at work, as if I must be nearing anorexia because I'm losing again. They hint that at home at night I'm viciously starving myself but this is far from the case. I'm much too much of a foodie and this is all about long-term rewards. I've always been good at the long game but have never applied it so single-mindedly to weight loss before.

ANOREXIA WAS HARDLY known about when I was at school. When I was about fourteen it suddenly flared up and a crop of wan troubled teenagers emerged. At my school they had to sit on the Anorexic Table at mealtimes, watched over by a firm teacher who policed them into eating. I remember girls who'd previously been healthy becoming suddenly paper-thin and white-faced, hiding pudding under their napkins and competing to eat less and less at every meal. It is extraordinary to remember that teachers once treated anorexia as a silly fad and a disciplinary matter.

Ten years after I left school, the death of Karen Carpenter changed all that. Suddenly anorexia was seen as a potential killer and therefore became a focus of attention. Over the years, the condition has become much better understood, but it remains very troubling. I've known a few sufferers. Most of them have won through in the end and returned to normal eating, but usually after a long and lonely struggle. I once worked with a girl called Leslie who was bulimic. She would ostentatiously eat big salads for lunch but still got thinner and thinner. She would sometimes smell slightly of sick and then disappear to brush her teeth. It was strangely distancing to guess what was going through her mind but feel completely unable to raise it with her.

Every now and then she would suddenly whack on a load of weight very quickly. I'm talking about stones piled on in only a week or so. When she let down her guard, she would explain that she was absolute. If she had one cake, she'd see no reason not to eat ten. The self-disgust of eating forbidden foods meant that all was lost and then she really might as well stuff her face. She was either rigidly self-controlled or dramatically out of control – there was nowhere in between.

Leslie didn't want to talk about her issues. She just desperately wanted to be thin at any price. Nothing else mattered and the rest of the world was frankly a distraction. At the same time she was excellent at her job. If I sometimes felt her soul was elsewhere, at least I knew her mind was safely occupied in work. Strangely enough, the bigger she was, the more outgoing and confident she seemed. But also, the unhappier she became.

Janine, another producer in the same company, was desperate to 'save' Leslie. She wanted to stage an intervention and get her 'seen' by someone. She felt we had a duty of care and that it was a full-on eating disorder. She was acting out of concern and friendship, but I couldn't agree.

I thought hard about her situation. I didn't think duty of care came into it. Was she an alcoholic, drinking and driving or getting into debt? No. Was she shooting up in the loos? No. Was she suicidal? No. Was she doing her job? Yes.

I cared about her very much but she was bright and intelligent and I believed in her. Most of all, I didn't want to patronise her. I have always hated to be patronised myself and I didn't want her to feel we were passing judgement on her. I felt she needed time to sort herself out, but she would do it.

My own food issues may have made me exactly the wrong person to work with her. I couldn't take a tough line with her, or indeed any sort of line. I empathised, but regarded her problem as her own private business, probably more strongly than someone who has never been beset by similar issues themselves. Or perhaps that was the right approach – at least it was respectful.

At the end of her contract, Leslie returned to London, where I think she went to therapy. I hope she found some peace with herself. I last heard from her when she had a baby, and was delighted to see her looking healthy and happy in the photos.

12st 6lb

Wednesday, 6 March 2013

LOSING DOESN'T CONTINUE at the same rate. The longest plateau in dieting history has struck again. I've been faithfully following the 5:2 diet, which served me so well at the start, but recently I've gone up and down the same two pounds every week for eleven weeks.

I'm size 14 and only a stone and a half overweight, but how annoying would it be to give up now? Today, when drying my hands on a tea towel, I pulled my rings off. It's official – they're too big, so I've decided that it's too dangerous to wear them. I'll lose them if I go on like this. I'm back to a bare hand for the time being. Every time I look at it I think, 'Soon I'll have them made smaller again. Soon.'

12st 6lb

End of March 2013

CHRIS BUYS ME chocolate for Easter, like a normal person. I'm not a big chocaholic and usually at Easter there's a kind of silent consensus that I had better not. But today I get a Turkish Delight (I have a weakness for them). I can't tell you what a vote of confidence this is. It's the closest to gushing he will ever be.

12st 4lb

Mid-April 2013

ONLY A COUPLE of months away from my two-year anniversary. How extraordinary is that. I fasted today, which was easy. I contemplated how far I've come. It's not so difficult any more. These days if I decide it's a fasting day, then it is. If I want to indulge, then I take a moment to decide that fully with my whole mind and intention – and then enjoy it.

〜

I haven't thought about Bridget for weeks, and have felt as if I'm struggling, despite a couple more pounds gone. I think of her now.

She's content, and is secure that the gains (losses) I've made will endure, but she's not so keen for me to lose more. She doesn't seem eager for change. She likes a default position.

Me, I'm full of plans and instigations, ready to move on. But I'll have to take her with me. Or vice versa.

〜

Our time scales are at odds, Bridget's and mine. She's the speedy one, intuitive, immediate. I am the book-keeper, recorder of the past, planner for the future, the strategist. No wonder we're at odds. 'I' in this scenario looks back with pain and forward with hopes and plans.

No wonder we don't see eye to eye. Unfortunately, she seems to have more control over instant decision-making. Like when she used to spur me on to grab a bag of nachos at the garage on the way home, for example. She can be a bit short-sighted like that. I don't do this any more, by the way, but still sometimes feel as if I could.

MEANWHILE, I WAKE in the middle of the night with excruciating leg cramps. I've had these symptoms before when travelling in hot countries for work. Taking an electrolyte solution cures the cramps but I'm worried about self-medicating. I see a doctor this morning to tell him about the cramps and mention the saga of my long diet.

He advises me to drink more water and increase salt in my diet (but not to excess). He reassures me that the electrolyte solution will do no harm, but suggests that I experiment with taking a tiny dose, which may well be enough to counter the effects of the diet. Then he begins to enthuse about my weight loss.

'But that's incredible, what you've achieved. You've probably put twenty years on your life. Obesity is a huge issue. Most people come in to see me and ask for a magic pill, they want to take something to just make it go away.'

Delighted with this vote of confidence, I ask if there is any intervention that the NHS can offer to help me to lose the last stone. It seems a reasonable request. I've lost over five stone without any help from them, so surely I'm due a bit of help? After all, as just pointed out, what I've done is a major exercise in disease prevention.

However, no joy. 'Sorry, but there's nothing we can teach you – if you've been dieting for two years you probably know more than we do! Just come back if your cramps cause you any more trouble.' He grins. I don't.

My friend Tina is a doctor. Later in the pub I complain to her about this response, which seems inadequate to say the least.

Tina is forthright. 'What do you want us to do? Chop your leg off?'

Shocked laughter.

'No, seriously, as a GP, no one's ever taught me about nutrition. How am I supposed to know anything about it?'

This is appalling. In any other circumstances, I would say, 'If true ...' but I know her, and there's no question but that she's telling it like it is. When the NHS spends such huge sums fixing the multitude of problems caused by poor nutrition, and the obesity that flows from it, how can dealing with it NOT be part of a GP's training? I'm incredulous.

Well that's that then. Back to Google.

12st 1lb

Mid-May 2014

HERE I AM, discontented because I still can't shift the last stone. This problem feels more technical than psychological at this stage (but note to self – who knows?). In other words, I'm sticking to my two fast days a week, plus moderate days in between, but can't seem to shift it. Have I gone into stasis?

The 5:2 diet has had great benefits over the six months I've followed it. As well as giving the pancreas a rest, it feels good for my overall well-being. I like the rhythm of cutting right back for two days and then being able to eat normally for the rest of the week. Once I've reached a BMI of 25 I may well return to this pattern as a way to live at ease with my weight, but for now that's enough. It's just not working well enough and I'm sure I can do better with another regime. Time to move on.

CHRIS HANDS ME an article tonight from one of the broadsheets about the mental problems of the obese. 'Overeating has a psychological element.' No!

'Having a gastric band won't work if you don't solve the eating disorder first.' Really?!

How on earth do people get paid actual money to write this stuff.

CHAPTER 23

Birthday honours

12st 4lb

Tuesday, 4 June 2013

What's Bridget up to? She's quite resolved. We don't seem to be fighting any more. She's working with me, not against me. She's a great reality check, which is ironic.

There was an embarrassing moment when I had to point out to her that my role, as 'system 2' brain, is to monitor and check her. Her decisions are based on a lot of automatic assumptions built up over years, but the job of our rational minds is to guide and update those assumptions. That's my bit.

I approached it carefully. If you remember, the last time I planned to do this she was in a paddy about who's in charge of willpower, so out of tact I ducked this subject. But I do need to talk to her about it.

Sitting on the moor one evening, I begin gently, 'You know I've always conceded that you're the decision-maker round here?'

She's not looking at me, is busy shoring up the banks of a small stream. She shrugs in agreement.

'Well, I've come across something else.'

She glances sharply at me and then casually resumes packing stones along the stream's edge. But I can tell she's listening.

'Apparently it's my job to make sure we're on the right track.' Carefully I say 'we' not 'you'.

'I have to work out if our strategy needs updating. Then of course it's up to you to put it into practice.'

It feels like telling your mum you're supposed to spy on her.

'I think we're on to a good system – don't you?' but she's gone. Disappeared. In the distance I see her striding into the woods.

It seems she doesn't do collaboration.

TODAY IS MY second anniversary and I've lost over five stone. In AA the start date of sobriety is celebrated each year with a birthday, often with cake. The person in recovery talks about their journey so far, family and friends come and bear witness to the positive outcome. By contrast mine today is quiet and reflective. Losing weight has more shame and privacy attached to it, perhaps.

At the beginning I committed to a year but with great trepidation. I couldn't imagine sticking to it, but I did. At the end of year one there was no question that I would give up. I feel the same again now. Stopping is not even on my radar.

Having come so far, I'm still struggling to achieve that elusive BMI 25. I'm looking for a new diet and am tempted to try a radical solution, perhaps meal replacement. I attend a sales meeting for one famous brand to test the waters. The group leader, Emily, is pretty, heavily made-up, slim and glamorous. I ask her if she's ever been on the diet. She prickles and sits up straight like a meercat.

'Why do you ask?' Defensive.

'I just wondered if you know what it feels like to live on such a low calorie diet, what it's like.'

'Well I've done it, of course I have.' Hollow laugh.

'I lost about two and half stone but then gradually one crept back on. I really need to get back on track. We all do it from time to time. What did you think – that we'd recommend something we're not doing ourselves?'

Why not? Everyone else does.

I ask for samples. It takes all my courage to replace my food with them for a day: one shake, one soup, one 'meal' – spaghetti bolognaise, but not as you know it, earthlings. It's astronaut food. In turns out to be bearable, if chemical tasting, and certainly not much like normal food.

It isn't the taste that puts me off so much as the fact that I actually disapprove of it. It's everything I've been working to avoid – quick, synthetic, extreme, not real food, anti-pleasure, won't teach me anything. Why would I do this? It feels like giving in to a gimmick.

What meal replacements promise is a very quick route to weight loss but the downside is said to be equally quick regain. Or if not, massive weight loss followed by a lot of loose skin. I know of one weight loss guru who shed eight stone in a year on a very low-calorie regime and was left with so much spare skin that the only option was surgery. Do it slowly enough and that doesn't happen. It seems I've already talked myself out of this one.

12st 3lb

Saturday, 8 June 2013

AFTER A LOT of conflicting advice, I finally settle on the Dukan diet. This regime is high protein, low fat, no fruit and limited vegetables. My body doesn't know what's hit it and I lose four pounds in week one.

I like the fact that Dr Dukan is a proper foodie, unlike a lot of diet gurus who seem to be borderline anti-food. His book is full of recipes and I try many of them: baked custards, diet mayo and lemon chicken, all in the first week. They are delicious and nearly (but not quite) sufficient compensation for missing out on fibre altogether.

The best discovery on this regime is diet yogurt. I'm not keen on diet foods in general, on the basis that they aren't much like food. I'd rather have a tiny portion of something real than more of something nasty. However, guided by this diet, I've tried them for the first time in years and I must admit they've come a long way. The diet is stringent about the percentage of fat and sugar they may contain, zero fat and preferably zero sugar/carb (there's a little flexibility on this, but definitely no more than 7 per cent). This is hard to source and I find myself standing for ten minutes at a time in the dairy aisle, reading labels.

I've already decided to ease up at the weekend. Breakfast with Chris and Orlando is a cornerstone of the week and the thought of it keeps me going while I spend a week packing home carb-free eggs and bacon for breakfast, smoked salmon and cottage cheese for lunch, and a large but entirely carb- and fat-free dinner. It's lavish, but to be honest, quickly becomes repetitive.

Early results are good and the weight loss is already notice-able; my colleagues once again amaze me with the speed at which they clock a few more pounds off. They are full of praise but I sense also a little wary. As I near the end of the journey, they're already anxious that I might go too far.

'You will tell me if I'm getting old and scrawny?' I thought this might reassure Anna.

'Nearly at that very place. But don't worry, I'll let you know when you're knocking on the door of saggy.'

'Thanks'.

11st 13lb

Saturday, 15 June 2013

THIS IS THE lightest I've been for over twenty-five years. Lighter than I was aged eighteen.

Chris runs regularly with the Hash House Harriers who make a weekly dash over the moors in the early evening. They meet at the same time all year round. In summer it's at twilight, glorious and golden, but in winter it's so dark you can't see your feet, pitch black. They run whatever the weather: rain, sleet, snow and fog.

Occasionally I go but always end up walking with those stragglers at the back whose knees have gone or who've had heart attacks or strokes so that gentle exercise is all they can do. I'm a fraud, bringing up the rear, because there's nothing actually wrong with me. There was more reason to lag behind when I carried five extra stone but now there's none. I could try harder, but so far have not.

My first attempt to run is stymied by lack of a sports bra. Never given it any thought, but it turns out to be an essential piece of equipment. Once kitted out, I try running gently but am breathless by ten metres. Gradually it gets easier, but to be honest never actually easy.

The mad thing is I'd assumed that because I've lost weight, I'd be able to keep up with the Hash. Not true, I still have to build up fitness. Over the next few days I get going. Soon I'm running a couple of miles twice a week and getting very slightly fitter.

THE DUKAN DIET is based on the idea that calories are not all equal. In other words, Dukan assumes 100 calories of sugar affects our weight in a fundamentally different way to 100 calories of lean meat. This is a red-hot issue in the world of dieting. The traditional advice has been the opposite: that 100 calories of cucumber counts the same as 100 calories of chocolate, and eating them will have exactly the same effect on your weight.

A calorie is the unit of energy it takes to raise the temperature of one gram of water by one degree Celsius. It's logical to assume that the whole point of this definition is to equalise the value and importance of one type of calorie with another. A school of thought known as CICO (calories in, calories out) adheres to this point of view and suggests it doesn't matter much what type of food you're eating because the overall calorie load is what counts. But that's exactly what is refuted by Dr Dukan.

He claims that the energy it takes to process food should be taken into account as it alters calorie uptake within the body. Protein is hardest to digest and takes most energy. For that reason, the first phase of the Dukan diet is almost pure protein for seven days and is therefore even stricter than the Atkins diet. It excludes all fruit and vegetables, which I find hard and somewhat counter-intuitive. However, I'm persisting.

Both the Dukan and Atkins diets aim to throw the body into 'ketosis', a fat-burning state which allegedly results in dramatic weight loss. In practice, both Atkins and Dukan turn out to be very low-calorie regimes. The reason is that the restrictions of these diets take away a lot of the pleasures of eating, so dieters naturally stop consuming sooner. They can eat as much lean protein as they want, but steak without chips has limited appeal, ditto eggs without toast.

One recent study showed that although initial weight loss is speedy on such diets, a broader-based low carb diet, including vegetables and fruit, had just as much success in the long run. Both improved blood sugar levels for diabetic and pre-diabetic patients. However, ketogenic diets also resulted in increased levels of LDL cholesterol, at least in the initial stages of the diet.

I've seen plenty of studies claiming the ketogenic diets are safe and promote long-term weight loss more effectively than other low carb diets. However, a study reported in the *American Journal of Clinical Nutrition* in 2006 examined whether the claims of 'metabolic advantage' was valid, and concluded that they were not.

So there we are – back to calories. Or at least, that is the case if you take the results of this one study to its logical conclusion: despite the claims of various diet gurus to the contrary, successful weight loss is actually achieved by calorie reduction, not by manipulation of body chemistry through eating certain 'approved' foods.

If obesity research and the diet industry are both still producing such contradictory advice on this issue, how are we mere dieters supposed to know what to think? Or what to eat for that matter.

NEARLY TWENTY YEARS ago I had a knee problem which wouldn't go away. It was diagnosed as a 'bucket-handled' tear which sounds like something Jack and Jill might have suffered, tumbling down that hill. To bring it up to date, it should be renamed a ring-pull tear because that's the shape of it, a curved sliver of cartilage which hooks on and locks the knee. Apparently it's common among young sportsmen and middle-aged overweight women. That's humiliating for a start.

The recommended treatment was keyhole surgery, still relatively new at that time. I was referred to a local orthopaedic surgeon. I checked him out and discovered that he had done the greatest number of these procedures locally and was highly thought of. Pre-op he came to see me on his ward round, surrounded by students.

'Might we have a quick look?'

'Yes of course,' I murmured.

'Now – here's a pretty kettle of fish. Look at this mass of subcutaneous fat. This is going to be quite tricky to plough through – extraordinary, look here, have a gander.'

I gritted my teeth as he rattled on. I weighed about fifteen stone at that time. Overweight, it's true, but there are many heavier people around. Why did he feel entitled to talk that way to my face? I was unusually silenced: I wanted him to do a good job and he did, despite having to wade his way through the 'mass' of subcutaneous fat. But how very rude.

Perhaps it's inevitable that doctors take a dim view of obesity given that it's a cause of multiple health problems. Presumably they see it as a form of self-harm. I'm trying to look at it from that surgeon's point of view, but it doesn't quite let him off the hook.

Knee surgery: 10.

Bedside manner: nil.

*

TWO MONTHS ON, I'm still in the second phase of the diet. Pure protein days are alternated with days of protein plus selected vegetables. There's advice to drink lots of water, which I do, but the very limited amount of fibre in my diet is really bothering me.

The F Plan diet, a leader in its day, was enthusiastic on the subject of poo. Audrey Eyton promoted a high fibre diet which she said would produce faeces that were 'soft and plentiful'. It was a relief that someone paid attention to this taboo subject. It is so often neglected by diet books, which is extraordinary as it is one of the predictable consequences of dieting. Later diets – Atkins, Dukan, South Beach, Grapefruit, Zone – are all low-calorie, low-carb diets with unpleasant side effects in this department. Why bring this up now? Let's just say I don't like everything about my new diet.

I should just mention that I've been forbidden by Chris to write about this topic, so here goes. He says, 'Too embarrassing, too easily sent up by unkind readers.' But I have faith and trust that my reader isn't unkind. It would be disingenuous to avoid it altogether. Every diet interrupts the normal flow and constipation is a regular side effect of many of them. Unlimited fruit and veg (within reason) are permitted on the WW plan and as they are high in fibre, they help keep everything moving even with a low calorie intake. Drinking lots of water is a big help, and both exercise and coffee have gentle laxative effects too.

Headlines to combat constipation are:

- Water
- Exercise
- Fruit and veg
- Wholegrains like porridge, wholemeal pasta and brown rice
- Coffee (but cautiously, because it increases insomnia and anxiety).

11st 11lb

Saturday, 10 August 2013

THE DUKAN DIET was great for a couple of months but the weight's not shifting substantially any more and I can't bear eating so few vegetables because it feels unhealthy. For me, the only way to avoid constipation on this diet is to take laxatives. Not a way to live. At the beginning it was appealing to eat as much protein as I liked, but even with good recipes the diet has quickly become repetitive and restrictive. Time to jump ship again. But what to? More research needed.

Before I leave it, there's one aspect of the Dukan diet that I really rate. It's the last phase of the diet – the Transition Phase. Dukan says that after weight loss, it takes five days per pound lost to reset your body to its new level. During that time you should eat a modest and regulated amount of carb and fat, gradually increasing as your body gets used to it. That would mean 440 days for me – around a year and a quarter. Perhaps a bit long, but the idea of a careful reintegration of normal eating makes sense to me. So many people lose, only to whack it all back on as soon as they relax their regime. I'm not going to do that.

I'm encouraged by an item on the radio claiming that Type 2 diabetes can be reversed by a very low-calorie diet. Well there, maybe I've done it – pushed away the shadow that hung over me when I started this journey. I would be very unlucky to get it now, even without losing those last nine pounds.

I may be repeating myself, because my brain sure is repeating itself. 'This isn't working, it's over, I'm done, I should give in and come quietly.' But I am sitting on a train where I have just eaten dinner. No starter, roast lamb, lots of carrots and broccoli. No bread, pudding, cheese or wine. I don't know where the decision came from to stick at it, but I am grateful, and I'm remembering to treat the doubts as white noise.

Every meal is another opportunity to slip not taken. Every meal is another small victory. Every meal is another chance to learn how to eat well.

SOME NIGHTS IT'S very tough indeed. I grumble and groan, to be met with seeming indifference by Chris and Orlando both. But on closer inspection, they're helping.

'Dad, will you go to the shop and get some chocolate?'

'Not tonight. She's had it tough today. I'm going without, doing what she's doing. Only with less fuss.'

They guffaw, but sympathetically.

I get the support under the laugh.

'And without the five-stone weight loss,' I add, just a little bit smug.

CHAPTER 24

See Saw Margery Daw

12st 4lb

Saturday, 21 December 2013

I'M BACK AT 12st 4lb. What can I say? It's infuriating, because I've been eating well. I don't know what's going on.

I've been summoned to see Bridget. Obviously there are no words involved (as if), but I know she wants to see me.

I labour up the hillside, under dark skies and rain, wondering what she wants. It's almost unheard of for her to communicate with me. Usually the boot is firmly on the other foot.

She has her back to me, sorting kindling for the fire, which is weak and sputtering, struggling to produce heat in this chilly atmosphere. I can feel a little tension in the air.

'What's the matter? Bridget?' She has turned away from me and is breaking sticks purposefully. To be honest I do have an inkling what this is about.

'You know that I've named this diary? I'm calling it The Fat Controller.'

This is not a question but a statement, because of course she knows everything that happens to me, and in fact much more than I'm conscious of.

'It's about controlling my weight ...' I'm stuttering like the fire, embarrassed. She does not meet my eye. 'Well yes it's also a play on words. It's about you too.'

I sense that I'm getting close to her issue.

'I'm not implying that you're fat.'

She nods curtly.

'Of course you're not fat.'

Suddenly I understand the problem. 'You've never had a weight issue, have you?'

No, she hasn't. She shakes her head, disdainful, and turns away.

BUT THIS IS extraordinary. If I accept that she's been controlling my eating all these years, how can this be? She's ensured that I was well-covered – why? Out of some obscure idea of what – protecting me? Maintaining the status quo? So why object so much at being thought fat herself? It doesn't make sense, until I realise that I myself have never really felt fat.

When people say to me now 'you must feel so much better' I disappoint them. I much prefer wearing size 14 to size 22, but that's about it. I was always energetic even when I carried an extra six stone.

Presumably I never felt fat because she never felt fat. In my inner self, I felt as though I was a normal weight. There are advantages: I wasn't filled with self-criticism even if I suffered the humiliations of obesity on the outside. But the disadvantages were greater: I wasn't sufficiently motivated to change and didn't fully realise how important it was that I did.

Perhaps that's why I've always hated photographs of myself: they never match my mental image of how I think I look. In my head I was a sort of middling weight, energetic, solid, but not vast – even when I was in fact clinically obese – so I reacted with shocked lack of recognition to photos. I would look at them and think, 'That's a really unfortunate angle.' It wasn't. It was what I looked like. I suffered from body dysmorphia the wrong way round – I thought I looked fine, and it was just photographs that made me look like a sack of potatoes.

All this flutters speedily through my mind. But I still need to make peace with Bridget.

'I guess that you'd rather I stick to my first idea, Two Light Years?'

Brisk nod.

'Even if, to be strictly accurate, it now needs to be Three and Half Light Years?'

I'm not sure, but I think she just rolled her eyes to heaven.

'Perhaps you'll get used to The Fat Controller.'

She turns her back to me again, a pretty clear indication that she won't get used to it. I'll have to give this one a bit more thought.

'THE 'APPESTAT' IS a word often used in concrete terms in the media to describe the body's natural mechanism for regulating its weight. It used to be a more popular phrase than it is now, but I still occasionally see references to it in articles like 'The appestat and binging: Why you can't eat just one' and 'How to recalibrate your appestat thermostat'. I begin to wonder why the word has fallen out of fashion so I look it up. The dictionary definition for it is 'a neural control centre within the hypothalamus of the brain that regulates the sense of hunger and satiety', which sounds oddly certain for something which is still the subject of some debate.

Noticing that it never appears in the studies I'm reading prompts me to look further. It turns out that the word 'appestat' was invented in the 1950s, the assumption being that regulation of weight was due to a single mechanism in the brain and that we would eventually find its location. Meanwhile it was named, but it's not a medical term.

GRACE KITTO

'I've never even heard of it. What is it?' said one doctor I asked.

The medical dictionary has a listing for it: 'a hypothetical region in the hypothalamus that is thought to regulate the appetite'. Note: hypothetical.

Why does this matter? Because it's one example of the way that speculation and hypothesis about weight control pass into language as certainty, spreading misinformation disguised as fact, very confusing to those of us at the coalface.

The current buzz phrase is the 'set point'. This is the idea that we have an internalised range of acceptable weights and the body uses all its tools to keep us there: hormones to respond to changing fat levels prompting hunger or fullness, motivating the behaviour changes which result in food actually going into our mouths. A similar idea to the putative appestat in fact, except the 'set point' theory focuses on the weight range itself rather than the mechanisms which achieve it.

In a TED talk entitled 'Why Dieting Doesn't Usually Work', neuroscientist Sandra Aamodt describes the set point as a range of ten to fifteen pounds within which the body naturally fluctuates. She says there are more than a dozen chemical signals in the brain telling us when to gain weight and another dozen telling us when to lose it. To guard against famine, when deprived of food, our brains send signals to slow metabolism in order to conserve resources. But in the modern world, with the easy availability of high calorie foods, this mechanism is bit of a curved ball. It makes it easier to gain weight and harder to lose it. According to Aamodt, the unkindest cut is the fact that the set point 'can go up but it rarely goes down'.

Aamodt herself gave up dieting as a New Year's resolution, lost ten pounds, and now considers it's the best thing she's ever done. All I would say is that looking at her now, it's clear she never was seriously overweight. *Fat is a Feminist Issue* carried a similar message, advising us to give up dieting, eat mindfully and let the weight find its own balance. This is great advice for anyone who is not clinically obese at the outset. For me there's a bit of counting to be done first, although the ultimate goal is the same: I too intend to give up dieting, but not till I'm done.

Unfortunately for us all, it seems that the body is predisposed to guard against weight loss more than to prevent weight gain. They call it an 'asymmetrical bias'. It's why people tend to put on weight as they get older – and also why it's harder to lose than to gain.

But not impossible. This note is from me, not from the studies. Not impossible.

OUR WORK CHRISTMAS lunch is always cheerful. This year we made a radical decision to hold it a few miles the other side of the Tamar Bridge, in Cornwall, in a spit and sawdust pub. We checked it out on a chilly Monday when the bar was bleak and empty, smelling of last night's beer, but the food was really good: scallops fresh from Looe Fish Market, swimming in garlic butter, and lovely goat's cheese salad. We took a plunge and booked it.

A week before Christmas all of us rocked up in a hired coach and poured in to find the pub transformed. There was a huge open fire with crackling logs and the wonderful welcoming scent of wood smoke. Green boughs of holly and mistletoe hung from low beams and along every windowsill. White fairy lights and occasional knots of red ribbon were dotted around. Beautiful. A perfect Dickensian scene.

As an antidote to the Christmas cheer, I wore black. I thought I looked fabulous, and indeed many people told me that I did, but my vision of myself was as slender as a girl. Looking at the photos later on I see a dumpy little figure, cheeks still plump, far from the sylph of my imagination. More a Queen Victoria of the middle years. But that's OK.

It's Bridget's fault. She persists in feeling that she doesn't have a weight problem. So my ambition now is to make what she feels is her natural size match my actual size. Then at last photographs will lose their power to pain and shock me.

I have lost no weight for four months. I am navigating through Christmas. It's fine.

WHEN WE MOVED to Devon in 2000 we took on a new mortgage. As part of the whole financial reappraisal, we took out a family insurance policy. We each attended a medical with a doctor appointed by the insurers. Neither of us drinks much or smokes so we were confident we'd get a clean bill of health.

The reports came back and as expected Chris's was fine. But mine said that because of my weight, my life expectancy was six and half years lower than average for my age. I was profoundly shocked, and made another huge effort on a crash diet which lasted all of five weeks. Then, as so often, it petered out. 'I've just got no willpower,' I told myself.

Willpower is such a loaded expression. Every woman I meet who frets about her extra pounds beats herself up for lack of willpower. This is the woman who gets her children to school, clean, fed and dressed on time, does a full day's work, shops, cleans the house, cooks, finds time to hear her children's stories of school friendships and break-ups, nature projects and apple pie competitions, baths them, kisses them, cuddles them, goes to bed, gets up and does it all again. Or if she doesn't have children, makes time for her friends, a social life, sports, evening classes, work, a life full of activities which fill every hour. She has willpower. That's not the issue.

Willpower suggests to me something done through gritted teeth, a reluctant submission of one's desires. There's something doomed to failure about it. In my own experience, a state of mind that has to be schooled, disciplined and held onto through clenched teeth is not sustainable. It's too hard, too energy-consuming. What I'm after is living at ease with Bridget, decisions fully made and committed to, loose hands on the bridle.

I want the force to be with me.

*

CHRIS HOLDS ME while I fret and fume about my beautiful, tragic sister Belinda, known as Bede. Thoughts of her consume me as I get closer to her weight. She died of a stroke nearly twenty years ago, aged only forty-seven, but I feel closer to her now than I have done for years.

I'm filled with anxieties and obscure feelings that being slim is not permitted to me. Bede broke away from our mother's conditioning to become more often thin than fat. My mother recruited me to her fat camp, even though I didn't want to be there. Now in some strange way I feel I'm moving between them, and am revealed, as if there's nowhere to hide. I am scared of who I am without my comfort blanket of fat around me.

Mind you, Bede wouldn't have approved of this account. Her weight yo-yoed, like mine, but only by a stone or two rather than the six-plus that I've been grappling with. She preferred to ignore it until it climbed to a level she couldn't bear and she would then live on cottage cheese for months until she got back to her desired level. The thinner, the better.

Feminism took off when I was in my teens and I was fired up by it. It helped shape me and showed me how to look at the world in a different way. Through feminist literature I became aware of the social pressure on women to be thin and felt increasingly conflicted about it as I grew into adulthood.

But if I talked to Bede about it, she would pooh-pooh it.

She'd say, 'Are you still going on about that?'

I'M NOT SLEEPING well. A curious thing has happened. I've started to find news reports unbearable. Any story of human suffering, especially violence, even more especially violence towards children, leaves me running the scene painfully through my mind, on a loop, in the middle of the night. I can't think where this has come from.

A seven-year-old boy in a blue jumper, beaten and bruised, catches my attention. The horror of his last moments, his small body abandoned, still alive. His bright face smiling on the news haunts me. I try various tricks to overcome the sorrow. In imagination, I wrap him in warm blankets and dab his wounds with soothing ointment. I speak softly to him. I honour him and feel his pain, trying to send him to sleep.

Only partially successful, I avoid news photography. The radio and broadsheets are all I can take. Which is more sane, to become numb to it, or to suffer so much you avoid it?

I haven't seen a therapist for years but now feels like a good time. A couple of weeks of rebalancing should put me back on track I think.

Footnote: don't worry about this child. He's a fiction, but he stands for all the real stories which left too many images in my head. I'm not serving any of them up here to fill your mind too. Not giving the real pain any more oxygen.

12st 2lbs

Tuesday, 14 January 2014

MOLLY AND I have a day in London in and out of meetings, no time to eat and anyway both trying not to overdo it. By six o'clock we're very peckish. We sit in a Fitzrovia hotel, waiting for the last appointment of the day, and order mint tea. It comes with chunky shortbread biscuits. We each eat one and then Molly takes a second one.

'I'm starving. Aren't you?'

'Yes I'm quite hungry.'

'Have another.'

'No thanks, I'll wait and have something proper to eat later.'

'Go on, have another – won't hurt, you've hardly eaten today.'

'No, it's OK, I'm fine now I've had one.'

Molly goes on pressing me, and then suddenly, without discussion, she stops a passing waitress in her tracks.

'Can you take these biscuits away please, they're tempting my friend. She doesn't want another one. They're looking at her!'

I laugh out loud. This is nothing to do with me. She must be talking about herself. Have I offended her by refusing a second biscuit? She would call it willpower, and both praise and blame me for it. 'You are good, you've got a will of iron' and 'Oh you're so hard on yourself, you could ease up occasionally.'

To me it feels like riding a bike. I'm in balance with this decision. I decided to eat one biscuit, so I did. Now I've decided not to eat another one, so I haven't. I'm not trying to be annoying.

CHAPTER 25

Page 3 or bust

11st 13lb

Friday, 14 February 2014

She's tending an acrid fire, smoke billowing across the tors.

'I thought I'd just check in,' I begin. 'I've come to the conclusion that I need to restrict even more how much I eat, unless I start to exercise more. I've nearly come to a complete standstill, what with Christmas and my birthday …'

She raises one bushy eyebrow and pokes her fire. I feel the need to reassure her about what I'm doing, as if she might be scared to let me carry on. This is crazy but I can only act on instinct. If called to reassure, then reassure.

'I'm not getting anorexic,' I say. 'Just trying to keep moving.'

I distinctly see a smirk in the form of a small quirk of the lip. She seems to be saying, 'Of course you're not – you're still twelve pounds overweight. Duh.'

'And I'm eating plenty of food.'

She glances at me seriously.

'Yes I am. I am not starving myself, nor will I.'

Brief nod. OK then. Proceed.

OUR CLEANERS AT work have been away for three months, visiting their daughter in New Zealand. I often work late and they arrive and roll out the hoovers just as I'm finishing up. They like to chat but of course I want to send one last email or two and then get home – so I'm sometimes a little distracted.

A few days after their return, I get up from my chair to leave and Bob barks, 'I thought so! Look at you – you've lost loads! 'Ere – Val, look. I wasn't sure, you sat there, but now you're standing up, I can see it plain as day. Cor bloody hell! You go on the way you're going, you're gonna be a Page Three girl!'

Small moments like this keep me going. A laugh, but I was moved too. I was never, under any circumstances, heading for Page Three* but he was being complimentary, and I got that.

THERAPY STARTS. I keep thinking it'll be short-lived, that I might leave soon. But I don't.

It's honest, hard work and healing.

I discover attitudes about my obesity that I had no idea I held. I knew that it felt protective but I didn't know that I associated it with warmth and approachability too. I didn't know that I feared being thin, was anxious that it would make me either aggressive or predatory. I had no idea where these beliefs sprang from but, through therapy, I was able to explore and understand them. Then was happy to wave them goodbye. Held up to the light, they had no substance, no energy.

Mental spring cleaning. Fresh, invigorating and, yes, healing.

The Men Who Made Us Fat is an excellent TV series which I've been catching up on. It claims that the insurance industry first popularised the concept of BMI in the forties. Through the 1990s BMI boundaries were revised and refined, and in 1998 the World Health Organization finally shifted them to their current levels. Overnight millions of perfectly healthy

---

* Historical note: Page 3 was a regular feature in *The Sun* showing topless girls on the third page of the newspaper. The feature ran for forty-five years solidly from 1970 but for three years from 2012 it was the subject of a campaign to stop it, on the grounds that it was degrading to women.

Americans were categorised as overweight. They were sold diet products that don't work, diet regimes that they became addicted to even though they also don't work, gym memberships when exercise isn't proven to work either ... you get the picture.

Since then, around the world, we've spent billions on diet and exercise programmes but we're still getting fatter. *The Men Who Made Us Fat* used population statistics as evidence that diets don't work. It was a clear and well-argued series, but after watching I was left with a problem. If you are seriously overweight, what in the name of heaven are you supposed to do – refuse to diet because the whole industry is a con? Surely that's not the answer.

In the last four decades, global obesity has nearly doubled. In Britain it's more than trebled. The NHS spends at least 10 per cent of its budget caring for people with Type 2 diabetes, including complications arising from the condition, totalling over £14 billion a year. Obesity can be debilitating and is likely to lead to ill health and early death. So although we may blame the diet industry for monetising the issue and promoting products which don't actually offer solutions, we do nevertheless need solutions. If the answers don't lie in paying large organisations to spoon-feed us diet goods, then we must look elsewhere. For me, that meant searching inside, not out, for answers.

Forty years I've been on this treadmill and I'm looking forward to the end of it. Until my early forties, a BMI of 27.3 was the top end of healthy for women, which on me would have been just under twelve stone. That's where I am now. If I could time travel, I would have reached my goal already. But gradually, after 1998, other bodies like the National Institutes of Health in the USA followed the WHO's reclassification. The NHS fell in line too, and yet even today its own online BMI calculator still suggests BMI 25 is healthy. In other words, over my lifetime the goal posts have subtly shifted. Much like dietary advice. And indeed like the physiological explanations for obesity. All change, all the time. But subtly, as if we might not notice.

I HAVEN'T SEEN my old school friend Naomi for over two years. The first thing she says is, 'Amazing! How did you do it?' And the second, 'Now I'm more scared of you than ever!'

And there you have it: women's ambivalence about body shape, their own and other people's. I didn't lose weight to offer anyone a threat, nor am I even approaching thin. Twelve stone may be what I weighed when I was eighteen but it's hardly fairy-like.

To be honest, there have been far more positive responses than negative ones to my new size and shape. Trouble is, the negative ones are more shocking, funnier and much more interesting – so there's a lot more to say about them.

WATCHING THE SERIES prompts me to re-read *Fat is a Feminist Issue*, one of the most influential books on the subject of weight loss since my twenties. It's been on my bookshelf for forty years, often dipped into, always illuminating. I pick it up to browse and find myself gripped, reading from beginning to end yet again, nodding at every page. Still relevant, still mould-breaking.

'Compulsive eaters crave their food as badly as a junkie craves heroin ... They are always going "cold turkey" – dieting or fasting – or trying their methadone substitute – cottage cheese.' I laugh in recognition at this, but it's a painful sort of laughter.

Susie Orbach's observations were based on women's testimonies collected in the context of support groups she ran, in which she was able to explore the issues of body image and gender. Disempowerment and abuse run through the text like seams of metal through rock. It is as moving and inspiring as on first reading. I was left wondering why, all those years ago, it didn't enable me overcome my food compulsions.

There's a crucial central message which it seems I've skittered over all these years, understanding it intellectually, but not emotionally. Susie Orbach describes six vital steps used to start work with a new group.

Step one: 'To demonstrate that the compulsive eater has an interest in being fat.' The words are simple but the meaning takes more time. It must logically be true. Why replicate behaviour that causes personal unhappiness and potential ill-health if not that we have competing motivations, in conflict with each other?

Step two: 'To show that this interest is largely unconscious.' I almost laugh out loud. No wonder I took this very question to Bridget, asking her to give up whatever her motivations are for keeping me fat. Finally, after forty years, I accept that this is true. I have had unconscious reasons for compulsive eating and weight gain. I am busy articulating those reasons and challenging them.

Right from the start, when I first read the book, I took to heart the idea that the ultimate goal was to give up both dieting and food obsession, letting my weight take care of itself and find its own healthy level. In my twenties I gave it a go, but my weight never did find that healthy balance.

Nearly three years into this current project, which actually I've decided to stop calling a diet, there is the beginning of a realisation as to why that was so. I understood parts of the argument, and embraced them, but ducked the parts that were too hard to confront. I've saved the hardest bits till last.

On this re-reading, I take the same message from the book that I did all those years ago but with a caveat: yes to giving up dieting and food obsession, but tempered with the need to actually shed obesity first. And if that sounds a little contradictory – it is.

Tina, my doctor friend, tells me that a BMI of 30–40 is common among her patients. It worries her that they can't see anything wrong with that. They obviously haven't read the statistics. I'm not giving in until I get to BMI 25. That'll do me fine.

I want to get to the point when I say, 'Enough is enough,' and can rest.

THERE'S NEWS THIS morning that as part of a response to the obesity crisis, bariatric surgery is going to be made more easily available.

The NHS website says, 'Obesity is a psychosocial and social burden, often resulting in social stigma, low self-esteem, reduced mobility and a generally poorer quality of life.' Well, yes, it can be.

But when it adds that patients have to commit to following a restricted eating plan and doing regular exercise after surgery, that's where I take issue. How can they commit to any such thing? Without the practice before surgery, how will they know what they may be capable of doing afterwards? Unless they do the mental work, I don't see what any such commitment would be worth. I certainly couldn't have done it without my own Bridget-run brain gym. And if you do the mental work, then the surgery isn't necessary.

Fix your heads people.

NO SOONER THOUGHT than challenged. My friend Bella comes to stay, dramatically five stone lighter than when I last saw her. She's had surgery and she's relieved and delighted at her sudden weight reduction. Many attempts to lose weight over the years had ended in failure and, at last, here's success.

'Of course I've got an apron,' she says, gesturing at her abdomen. 'I'll have to have a tuck or two.' Apparently her loose skin won't shrink back but will have to be surgically removed.

'I feel as though I've cheated. I haven't done it like you. Mine was a short cut. You did it properly.'

I deny it, but guiltily realise that she's voiced my own prejudice. Seeing her in front of me, healthy and happy, the moral high ground crumbles away under me. It's obvious that from her point of view this is a much better solution than living with misery-inducing and debilitating obesity.

But should surgery really be provided more widely at the expense of the NHS? Apparently the obesity crisis is set to cripple health services in the western world so the temptation is for policy makers to seize on it as a solution. Less invasive methods of weight control, like therapy, so the argument goes, are potentially more expensive and may be slower to deliver success.

We need more research into causality, more techniques to deal with weight issues which might include surgery, but not be limited to it. If we really are in the middle of an obesity crisis, then surely we need to explore the problem much more widely for the long term. Surgery might be a quick fix and a short-term solution, but there must be better and more enduring ways of tackling obesity.

THERE'S A PICTURE spread in the weekend papers about a woman who lost half her bodyweight in a year. She is a photographer and she recorded images of herself before and after her weight loss. More articles about her appear in magazines and online over succeeding weeks. Two lines of argument run through most of them:

1. Her photographs are as repulsive as they are beautiful.
2. She's lost all this weight – and she's still not happy.

The pictures are works of art which celebrate her individuality and her life. They are extraordinarily confident and controlled. She looks entirely present in them. The first set was taken before she lost a pound. She knew exactly what she was recording and why.

If she were photographing someone else it might feel like a freak show, but the very fact that she's making images of her own body makes a crucial difference and gives the pictures a particular impact and poignancy.

She's lost weight in a completely different way to me, quick and dramatic. She exercised to the max and lost ten stone in a year, halving her body weight. Given the speed of her diet, it's not surprising that her skin is a little loose. The reporter seems torn between a longing to know exactly how she did it (less food, lots of exercise), repulsion at her 'before' body and a triumphant cry that even after all that weight loss, she's still not content!

Well why would she be? The theory is that we eat for comfort and to block out bad feelings. By that logic, reducing calorie intake on a dramatic scale means losing the source of comfort and bumping up against some of those negative feelings. She'll have to learn new ways to seek solace. Reading her interview, it sounds as though she's well aware of that.

Losing weight does not per se make us happy. It's a nonsense to think that it would. What it can do is to remove one big source of unhappiness i.e. the weight – as well as a source of consolation i.e. the food.

So what are we left with? A different set of problems. But what can you do? You don't want problems, don't be human.

I TELL STORIES in therapy, lots of stories. When asked about my feelings, inevitably my answers start, 'I think—'

'But what do you feel?'

'I don't know.'

Thinking has got me out of a lot of tricky situations. It's my first port of call. It's what I rely on.

PARTLY INSPIRED BY the photographer who halved her weight, I decide that at last the time has come to really increase my activity levels. Exercise burns only a small number of calories considering the effort it takes, but numerous sources confidently inform me that it will also boost my metabolism. I am doubtful, but I've come to accept that it's time I threw myself at it.

What is less controversial is that exercise improves overall fitness. A cardiovascular workout increases heart health, and some say that we should all get out of breath at least once a day. None of this can be bad.

This is still not about love of exercise for its own sake of course, so I want to target my efforts for maximum efficiency. At my request, Chris gave me a pedometer for Christmas. He asked me to choose it for myself because there are so many on the market, all so complicated. Some come as satellite wristbands which plot the distance covered when you run and then upload your speed and distance automatically to a website.

For those targeted at weight loss, rather than fitness, the mass of products around is equally impenetrable. My least favourite is one which allows you to earn Piggy Points (let's call them that) to be eaten as food. But I don't want to add yet another system of counting to my programme.

Despite having put the programme on the back burner for now, I chose a WW pedometer. It's out of the ark in that it doesn't track or automatically upload anything to anywhere. Fine by me. The first shock is that I have to walk 10,000 steps before it goes into 'earning' mode. Then walk more to earn each point. It would be good to share with you how many steps per point but the instructions here are obscure: 'This will be totally unique to you and as it will depend on your weight and stride length, it will vary for each individual.'

The very day after I got it, in the first flush of enthusiasm, I decided to put some serious effort into running by starting with our local Jingle Bell Jog around Burrator Reservoir on Boxing Day. It consisted of a four-mile loop skirting the water, and it took me more than fifty-five minutes to complete. Everyone else was long done by the time I got to the finish line. I was exhausted, but proud to have kept going for the whole distance, even if in slow motion.

Over the next few weeks I try to make friends with my new pedometer. The goal is to earn 14 points per week. That's a lot of exercise on top of 10,000 steps a day that you're supposed to be walking anyway, just to reach par. I manage to earn one to two points about three times a week. The rest of the time I struggle to reach baseline activity level. So part of the problem is that I'm just not active enough. This is useful information and at least having the pedometer has helped me to see it.

Having started, I join Chris for another evening run with the Hash and am moderately successful. I'm not walking any more, but gently running.

On my fourth run since this new spurt of energy my confidence is building. I team up with another newbie, get chatting and somehow, between us, we manage to get thoroughly lost on a high stretch of moorland. Her phone battery has already packed up. Classic schoolgirl error, I think, confident in my own phone.

I'm loath to call Chris because it feels ridiculous – we're so near home, we're sure to pick up the trail any minute. We can see the lights of Plymouth in the distance so we know which way is south, we'll be fine. We walk to and fro, again and again across the same piece of ground, desperately trying to orientate ourselves, but we can't find our way down. It's hopeless.

The night is very clear, dark and starry, and there are animals everywhere – sheep, cows and horses. Stumbling over rough ground, a loud 'moo' in my left ear makes us both jump. We aren't really scared, though. We're sure we'll work out where we are soon. We don't.

I give in and call Chris, who's already in the pub. 'Where are you?' he sounds bored, but I know him and can sense his worry underneath.

'Well, not sure but I think—' At that moment, my phone cuts out too. Battery totally kaput. Whoops. Classic schoolgirl error number two.

Now our troubles have notched up a gear. Many of the Hashers volunteer for Dartmoor Rescue and as soon as they realise we really are lost, we know they'll come looking for us

– but I burn up with shame. After a run, all anyone wants is a quiet drink in the pub, not a scramble through bracken to find a couple of lost sheep like us.

On the very top of this particular tor is a rocky outcrop. It looks uncannily like my imagined home for Bridget. I have the surreal experience of life imitating art. Bridget's home is her cave high on the moors, and here I am, wandering around lost, stumbling among huge rocks in the velvety dark, surrounded by animal noises. I am very glad to have friendly company or I might have been spooked.

Nearly an hour later, to our great relief, a beam of torchlight comes slanting and bobbing across the fields. We are helped over a barbed wire fence, across two fields and a ditch into a waiting Land Rover and back to the pub. In company we put a brave face on it but at home in bed I can't stop trembling. Delayed shock I think.

It turns out that we were found at Shaugh Beacon, halfway to Cadover Bridge.

Was Bridget having a laugh?

Sobering fact #22: *A group of 105 women who received cognitive therapy lost more weight and kept it off over the next 18 months, while those assigned to a waiting list for therapy gained weight over the same period.*

Journal of Eating and Weight Disorders, 2005

CHAPTER 26

Denial is not just a river in Egypt

Saturday, 31 May 2014

Five stone lighter, it's less of a struggle to get up to Bridget's eyrie these days. I still approach respectfully.

She gives a brief nod. I sit by her fire and watch her cook; she seems to be baking herself some fish over an open fire. It's filleted, stretched out and threaded onto lengths of sapling which she's turning in the flames. I feel honoured. This is the first time I've seen her eat. Perhaps she thinks it's safe to show me food now because I'm in balance with my own diet so it won't give me dodgy ideas.

It turns out that she eats sparingly and well. Of course she does. (I could add – why then did she subject me to so many huge meals over the years? But perhaps that's churlish.)

'What do I do about misery, Bridget?' I ask.

She grins wolfishly. I know she's smirking at all those diet adages: don't eat your way through pain, feel it. Don't use food to anaesthetise yourself, let the feelings flow.

'It's all very well to laugh at all that homespun hokum, but what do I do instead of numbing myself with nachos? What does it actually mean – "feel it"? "Experience it"? Eating cake didn't stop me doing that. It just added a layer of guilt on top of the bad feelings I already had. What am I supposed to do to make myself feel better?'

She looks serious suddenly and gazes at her fish with deep interest.

'Ah I see. The universe doesn't actually give a monkey's whether I feel better or not. So the message is – deal with it myself. Work on the positive. Don't just try not to feel bad, work out how to feel better?'

She hands me a piece of fish, perfectly cooked, almost smoked, succulent and soft, and takes my breath away with this one simple act. I laugh out loud – 'But surely you're rewarding me with food? That can't be right?'

SINCE RE-READING *Fat is a Feminist Issue*, I'm increasingly uncomfortable recording my weight at every opportunity. I'm still committed to the overall goal but need to prune as much of the obsessive behaviour around food that I can.

I've been the same weight for over a year, still about 10 pounds over a BMI of 25, but stable. You could say I've been learning to maintain a healthy weight. Or you could say I've nearly achieved my goal, but not quite. Is it really obsessive of me to continue the hunt for that elusive BMI of 25? Yes, somewhat.

There are critics of BMI used as a measure of healthy weight. It's true that a person with a lot of muscle may have a BMI in the overweight category, despite being fit, since muscle weighs more than fat. They point out that BMI is a 'one size fits all' scale which takes no account of muscle mass, frame size, bone density or distribution of fat.

Waist measurement is thought by some to be a better indicator of the prospect for future health than normal range BMI because it indicates when the body is holding fat around vital organs. You are supposed to take your height in inches and halve it. For example, I'm five foot six so according to this advice, my waist should measure thirty-three inches. It is in fact thirty-four inches, not far off.

For me, as it happens, the BMI scale works well. I can understand the problems with it but I'm not particularly muscly, so that's not an issue. There's a wide spectrum of weights classified as healthy for my height, from 8st 13lb to 11st 2lb. The top end of that scale works for me, or I think it would if only I could get there.

I WOKE UP today with a headache, freezing as usual. I've been cold for months. I make about three hot water bottles a day. Living in an Edwardian house on Dartmoor, with wind blowing under the tiles, the east wind creeping round the corners of the house and the wettest, windiest winter, followed by the coldest, dampest spring for years, it's hardly surprising. We have an open fire in the evening, watch sitcoms together and huddle.

Chris says he'll build me a green passive house to keep me warm in our old age.

'It's probably because you've lost so much weight that you're feeling the cold so badly.'

Am totally taken aback – of course. Why had that never occurred to me?

IF I COULD bear the cold, it would actually be beneficial not to turn to a hot water bottle. It takes calories to keep warm and staying cool prompts our fat cells to generate heat. This theory has been tested and offers yet another way to revolutionise weight loss.

Fat in the body has always been described as falling into two categories, 'brown' fat, which generates heat and is a power source around vital organs, and 'white' fat, which generates love handles.

Now scientists have discovered what they are calling 'beige' fat. This occurs when white fat gets very cold, at which point it has the ability to generate some heat, but less than brown fat – hence the unprepossessing name.

Researchers at the University of Kentucky School of Medicine strapped cold packs to specific areas of white fat on the thighs for thirty minutes at a time. At the end of that time they tested the thigh fat again and found three genetic markers for beige fat. They are cautiously optimistic that this technique will lead to a breakthrough.

Other studies have shown that belly fat biopsied in winter shows more genetic markers for beige fat than in summer, as we use calories to battle the cold. This explains why our diet is naturally inclined towards fatty foods in winter. Ask an Icelander – they eat butter, blubber and oily fish in profusion. It suits the climate.

The bad news, though, is that in obese people white fat was less likely to turn beige. 'Our findings indicate inflammation can hinder the conversion of white to beige fat,' said Dr Philip Kern, one of the study authors.

Another simple technique to aid weight loss is to turn our household heating down. Most of us set it at around 21–22°C but a study at Maastricht University Medical Centre found that reducing household heating to 15–17°C for several hours a day promotes healthy weight.

Note to self: put the hot water bottle down. Now.

Wednesday, 4 June 2014

MY THIRD DIET birthday and I'm still in roughly the same place, with minor ups and downs, which is both good and bad.

It's a Saturday, relaxed, sociable and cheerful – and then suddenly, bam, I'm completely off course: I end up eating about 2500 calories of random food, including a whole packet of butterscotch Angel Delight, a throwback to the Fray Bentos pie years. I haven't tasted it for thirty years and won't for another thirty. Now feel stuffed and slightly anxious, but the point is that this is actually OK. I am still only 12st 4lb. I will sort it out tomorrow. Years of food anxiety are hard to get over, but I've finally learned I can rely on myself to pull back when I need to.

Fat is a Feminist Issue makes the point that many women become their own internal police force, monitoring and disciplining themselves over their intake, lacking trust in their errant and treacherous bodies. Too true.

What this latest episode tells me is that I will probably always have moments of uncontrolled eating. If I learn to live with them and work around them, there'll be no harm done. I hope that as time goes by they'll become rarer, but if they don't, so be it. They may never disappear completely. I'm at peace with that.

YEARS AGO I was having supper with some friends in Bristol. Pip was at the head of the table. He'd been reading Wittgenstein and was blown away. When Wittgenstein was asked, 'What is the aim of your philosophy?' he answered, 'To show the fly the way out of the bottle.' Pip was intrigued by this answer and asked me what I thought it meant.

'If you imagine a fly in a bottle, how do you get it out?' he said. I realised he wanted me to work it out, then and there.

'Can you break the bottle?' I asked.

'No. You can't use suction, or cut it, or melt it. You just have to work it out.'

'Oh I see,' I began to laugh. 'That's very clever.'

He was impressed, but doubtful, wanted to know whether I had really got it.

'Excuse me,' he said, very polite, and I was conscious of the six people around the table listening, 'but do you mind telling me what you think the answer is?'

'Well the fly's already out of the bottle. I've done it. I just had to imagine it out, and the thing was done.'

That was more than thirty years ago. A small moment of glory at a dinner table. I could work out a problem that didn't matter as a party trick, but for two decades more I have failed to apply that lesson to my own life.

But now I think I've got it. I've seen the light. You just have to imagine the fly out of the bottle, and it's out.

*

THIS EVENING I had a long conversation with my brother Crispin about the nature of addiction. After all this time, I found myself telling him about the row with Chris, when he compared me to an alcoholic.

'It was ridiculous,' I said.

'Why?' my brother asked.

'Because I don't have an addictive personality. I've never drunk, or smoked, or taken drugs. It's just not me.'

'How would you define addiction?' he said.

'Well, compulsive behaviour. A habit. Something you're driven to do despite yourself, overriding rational thought.'

'Uh-huh.'

'Oh.'

It's rare that you can pinpoint the moment when your opinion shifted and you suddenly saw something you had been blind to before, but here's an instance. Up till this point I was completely sure that Chris's analogy with alcoholism was both wrong-headed and offensive. By the end of our phone call, the scales had fallen from my eyes and I realised that my behaviour has always had all the hallmarks of addiction.

It's helpful to know. When I go a bit bonkers around food at least I'll know what I'm dealing with.

I hate to say this, but Chris – you were right. And you know better than anyone what it costs me to admit that.

THE NEWS IS still full of the obesity crisis. Every morning I have the sensation that John Humphrys is addressing me personally. But how could he be? I'm not obese any more. Then again, when I was obese I didn't recognise it either. I hid from it, denied it, didn't want to see it. Now I've got the opposite problem. I still identify as obese even though I'm not.

If this whole project has taught me anything, it is to take my assumptions with a big pinch of best sea salt, hold them up to the light and reconsider. Just to mix a metaphor or two.

Huge figures are being bandied about: the number of obese

adults, the number of deaths from obesity-related conditions, childhood diabetes rates. Politicians speculate on causes. I read these articles wearily. They are too often full of shallow received wisdom.

John Humphrys is interviewing the Health Secretary, busy declaring that obese adults are those who have not learned to 'self soothe' in childhood so they turn to food for comfort. Really? All of them? Another glib hypothesis.

No mention of the role of the food industry here, you note. While the physiological reasons for obesity are so partially understood, this sounds to me like a sweeping generalisation which once more puts all responsibility straight onto us failing fatties.

The idea of Bridget is soothing in a way. You could certainly say she's a soothsayer. She offers no platitudes. But she understands what passes through my brain better than I do, accepts everything I do, and shows me the truth. That's the most self-soothing thing I can think of.

Sobering fact #23: *In the UK, about £6 billion a year is spent on the direct medical costs of conditions related to being overweight or obese in addition to the cost of diabetes care.*

McKinsey & Company, 2014

CHAPTER 27

Slippery scales

Saturday, 2 August 2014

I stomp up to the moor with a right old cob on.

'Can you believe what I've done?'

She can.

'How could I have been so stupid? Who was I fooling?'

Today I weighed myself on Maggie's scales and realised that mine are calibrated wrongly. Maggie has just checked hers with the ones at the surgery and they're accurate. Years ago I thought mine overweighed by four pounds and so, at the beginning of my diet, I adjusted them. To match them, I set the scales in the other bathroom at zero minus four pounds too. That means every weight I've recorded since is four pounds out. This is self-delusion in a big way. What was I thinking?

Now I've set both sets of scales back to zero. The result is that where yesterday they read 12st 4lb, today reads as 12st 8lb. Painful, but must be done to restore truth to these proceedings.

She doesn't meet my eye. Suddenly it dawns on me. She knew all along.

'Bridget! You did it. You kidded me into thinking my scales were overweighing. You made me adjust them in the first place.'

A slow grin. She doesn't even deny it.

'What did you think that would achieve? It was never going to last.'

She looks secretive, and mischievous.

'You knew I'd work it out eventually … but you thought it would keep me encouraged early on? I suppose that's true.'

I'm reluctant to admit this. I feel like an idiot for being taken in, but at least I begin to see what she was about. Perhaps she had my best interests at heart.

The point is that I knew I had adjusted those scales. How much denial was in that act? I can't blame Bridget for everything.

⁓

SUGAR IS THE new bad guy in town: nutrient-free, tooth-rotting, diabetes-producing, fattening, massively addictive sugar. All this we know, but now it's being described as an analgesic too – basically, a painkiller. Babies fed sugar cried less than babies who were not. So that means there is a scientific basis to the idea of comfort eating. It means you really can eat so as not to feel, feeding to get numb.

It's a strangely disconcerting idea. I can cope with the thought that we are psychologically dependent on food, but if the comfort is actually in the physical dimension that means sugar really does act like a narcotic. I've referred before to 'narcotic eating', perhaps closer to the truth than I imagined.

At the moment I'm trying juicing. Yesterday was a fasting day, juice only. I was hungry but focused. At lunchtime I bumped into Gilly in the kitchen at work and while we stood chatting, she took a tub of coriander hummus out of the fridge for lunch, tasted it and said, 'That's amazing!'

It was so good she wanted me to try a little on the tip of a teaspoon. In that particular moment it would have been ridiculous to refuse it, so I didn't. She was right – it was absolutely lovely, but even that almost homeopathic quantity of food made it much more difficult afterwards to accept that I wasn't going to eat any more until evening.

All three of us, Chris, Orlando and I, have made radical changes to our diets since I started losing weight. Once upon a time I would peel twelve potatoes to make roast dinner for the three of us where now it's six. These days we weigh dried pasta rather than just chucking in half a packet. And we used to have rice, naan and poppadums with curry, but now we skip the rice and give the poppadums to the dog, who adores them. She runs round the kitchen snapping them up, as if they might escape.

ON THE HUNT for a new regime, I've been exploring the latest trend, which attacks both low fat foods and calorie counting as 'the greatest diet myths of our time'. *Escape the Diet Trap* by Dr John Briffa argues that a low fat diet inevitably leads to an increase in carbohydrate consumption because, as we know, carbs are used to make fat-free products palatable. He says a carb-rich diet leads to insulin resistance, which in turn is a cause of Type 2 diabetes. I read his book in a single sitting. I'm thoroughly boggled because these ideas turn everything I thought I knew about dieting completely on its head.

Low fat has held sway since the 1960s but an increasing number of critics have observed that the big surge in obesity in developed countries dates from exactly that time. They're now asking whether there's a direct causal link.

For the last fifty years most advice for losing weight has focused on reducing calorie intake. Fat is calorie dense, so out it goes, according to this model of dieting. But *Escape the Diet Trap* argues that carbs are the real problem, as indeed our ancestors believed for hundreds of years before the low fat revolution. Crucially, as Dr Dukan also observed, the amount of energy it takes to metabolise different types of foods varies. Carbohydrates provide energy almost immediately whereas fats have to go through several more stages of oxidisation before they become available as energy. Dr Briffa therefore suggests that we radically reduce carbohydrates in our diet, replacing them with more fat and protein, which in turn will reduce insulin resistance and aid weight loss.

These arguments are completely new to me and they make my head spin. It's the total opposite of all the dietary advice I've been brought up on. Immediately I re-read the book to check that I've understood it. I have. Second time around it's still persuasive but I'm flummoxed. It's hard to believe. Am I brave enough to throw out the orthodoxy of the last few decades and try it? Of course I am.

I move on to a very low-carb regime of about 1200 calories per day, with a single slice of bread as my only major source of carbohydrate each day. It didn't feel as though it could possibly work but today I've shifted a few more pounds.

Between meals, the diet recommends occasional snacking on a handful of nuts and a piece of cheese. This combination quickly becomes a family favourite. Nuts are calorie rich, and on a low fat diet it would be unthinkable to eat so many at once. A small bag of cashews is 550 calories and the equivalent in carbohydrates would undoubtedly have caused me to gain weight overnight. It's immediately noticeable that the nuts don't have any effect on the scales in the morning.

Still shocked at this new anti-carb (and by extension, pro-fat) stance, I look for more literature. Gary Taubes has written persuasively in the same vein. In *Why We Get Fat* he presents the view that too many carbohydrates in our diets stimulate insulin secretion, which prompts us to store fat. Again, compelling reading.

This is why the Health Secretary should look beyond the personal for the causes of the obesity crisis. There are several candidates who should be held to account and made to change their ways: to name just two, the food industry for sneaking hidden sugar and salt into processed foods and the diet industry for sneaking hidden carbs into low fat foods. The Health Secretary should be concerned about these issues. The results, in terms of obesity, exercise huge pressures on the NHS. Loose talk about comfort eating is not the answer.

TRYING TO UNDERSTAND the science behind the causes of obesity and the routes to weight loss has become a kind of hobby.

It's fun to face the urge to eat with a barrage of internal questions. 'Now, am I stressed – is that cortisol secretion taking its toll? Too much ghrelin? Too little leptin? Or is it lack of sleep? Sleep is in fact a big candidate as I love the still small hours of the night. My favourite time for writing is when the house is quiet and everyone else is in bed. I also work full-time so that means I'm often sleep-deprived. It seems my own particular candle was designed to be burned at both ends. But as we know, sleep obesity is a thing. Note to self: try to sleep for at least seven hours a night.

How much help do these questions actually offer? Actually, a lot. When I began this project, as you know, magazine articles offering vague advice about comfort eating irritated me because they didn't ring true with my experience. But these days I can easily identify the cause of the stress, whether tiredness, thirst or overwork, and trace the effect on my hunger. Information is power.

What I'm always more reluctant to do is to look at the emotional reasons for overeating. And that, of course, is what therapy is for.

Monday, 4 August 2014

TODAY I LEFT home for London while it was still almost dark, only just dawn, heading into a long day. As I drove across the moor sheep were still clustered under the trees, huddling for warmth, the first streaks of light framing their woolly backs with a golden halo.

It was a very productive day and on the way home I was pleased to get to Paddington in plenty of time for the six o'clock to Plymouth. My train was announced and I followed a stream of passengers on to it and settled down for the three and a half hour journey back to Devon. We slid out of the station and the announcer welcomed us aboard the 18.03 – to Bristol. Wrong train.

Shocked and furious with myself, my eyes stung with held-back tears of frustration. I worked out quickly that there was just a chance I could swap trains at Reading and reroute home. But with only a minute's gap between the scheduled departure times of the two trains from Reading, I would have to leg it across the station to get to the right platform in time.

Other passengers helped me to position myself so I'd be right next to the escalators when we pulled in to Reading station. It worked, and I ran to catch the Plymouth train full of hope – immediately dashed when I reached the platform, panting, just in time to see it pull away and rumble off out of the station.

It was bitterly cold and windy and I had an hour to wait till the next train. I could have cried. At once my thoughts turned to food. I had had a good steady day, eating sensibly despite the challenges of the train travel offerings. Now I was really hungry but what struck me was the speed of my first thought, 'I could just go to that bakery and grab a Chelsea bun and a coffee. That would make me feel better.' But I knew that it wouldn't.

The difference between this temptation and the ice cream at Cadover Bridge is that I recognised what I was feeling before I acted on it. I felt desperate, hugely frustrated and with no one to blame but myself – I hadn't even checked which train I was getting on at Paddington. I do that journey so often, I really shouldn't have got it wrong. What a blasted idiot. But food was not the way to go. I had already bought a well-judged salmon salad for the journey home and decided to wait till I was at last on the right train before eating it. I drank coffee, walked around, snivelled a bit then settled down in patience.

Rattling about in my head was a small burble of comforting thoughts. 'You were tired,' I told myself. 'You made an easy mistake. It looked like that was your train, you followed the crowd onto a platform you'd normally expect yours to be on, it didn't take a second to get it wrong. You're hungry and you've been in balance all day, now you long to break your regime for comfort. But you know very well that if you do, at the other side of that Chelsea bun will just be the urge for something else. Pointless. Sit it out.' And so I did.

It took a person full of insight and compassion to point out to me later that this was self-soothing of a most positive kind. I hadn't realised it, but it's true. And it was exhilarating to realise that I've made a gap between tumultuous feelings and the drive to eat. For most of my life I've been so blind to those feelings that I've eaten before I was even aware where the urge came from. It was good to recognise the speed of the thought process – I feel bad, let's eat sugar. Recognising before doing gave me a choice about how to act, the very choice that was missing three years ago at Cadover Bridge.

DISCUSSING THAT MOMENT of choice with Chris, I find myself describing the thought of the Chelsea bun as a 'romance', an odd word, I know, but it seems to sum up the illusion wrapped up in the thought that eating will make me feel better.

Experience shows it will ultimately make me feel worse, and yet I continue to repeat the behaviour. Experience also shows that if I eat, while I am eating, I feel momentarily cheered, warmed, comforted, but almost the minute the food is finished, the same feelings of need and emptiness come back. This has happened time and time again. I know it, and yet the idea persists.

As I describe it, my eyes mist because I'm giving up this flimsy fantasy. It has no substance, but letting go of it is a small bereavement, a loss of sorts. And yet once I see it has no truth, what else is there but to name it as the sham it is?

I realise I've heard this story many times over from alcoholics who have had to give up the romance of the bottle, which also promises to make life easier, better, more fun – and never, ever delivers.

LAST NIGHT I met a friendly neighbour at a party. I've known her at a distance for a long time. Jenny is a clinical psychologist who works within an eating disorder programme. Apparently, our local city, Plymouth, is one of the fattest in the country. Nothing to do with me, I hasten to add. I was obese for many years before I moved here.

Jenny hasn't seen me in months and exclaims at my newly trim appearance.

'Very good. How did you do it?'

I'm struck by her sensitive praise, measured but affirming. I describe some of my techniques and because she seems really interested, go on to tell her, a bit shyly, about Bridget.

'So she doesn't answer when you ask her questions? Like a good therapist? Psychodynamic.'

'Except that it's inside my own mind. As though, if I look hard enough, the answers are all there.'

'Yes. They probably are. Sounds like what we call the "ancient mind". Or maybe like a shaman.'

'Other people have said that.'

She went on to tell me about some new work she's doing on trans-diagnostic therapy, which means, in simple terms, treating anorexics and obesenics as though they have the same disorder. It makes complete sense to me. I've known several anorexics with whom I've had a fellow feeling. We seem to understand instinctively that we're in the same camp.

'Obese people would be anorexics if they could, and anorexics fear they would be obese if they didn't control themselves so rigidly,' she said.

When we get home I report this conversation to Chris, with embellishments.

'So I'm a failed anorexic. No surprise really.'

'Not so failed, my love. Pretty triumphant in fact.'

I think my hearing is going.

MY SISTER JULIA and my step-sister Mandy have come to stay for the weekend. They both look me up and down, and I can tell they're really pleased for me. Julia smiles at me across the dining table and, for the first time, actually mentions my weight loss.

'You look like someone I used to know forty years ago,' she says.

'When did you start to notice I was losing?'

'Oh a long time ago. But sometimes in the past I've seen you after a gap and been shocked at how much you'd put on, because of the health implications. So I suppose I've learned to say nothing. And anyway, after a few minutes' natter you were what you've always been – my beautiful sister whose company I love.'

This is such a fair point, and so very kindly put, that I'm gob-smacked. Another eye-opener.

I can't have it both ways: I wouldn't have wanted her to tell me every time I had gained, so she learned not to keep up a running commentary. So reasonable. There are still surprises around every corner.

She's been saving up something to share with me.

'Did you know your birth weight was ten pounds?' she asks. I do. Ten and a half pounds.

'I've always wondered if mum's pregnancy with you was diabetic, because the rest of us were much lighter at birth – around seven to eight pounds, which is more normal.'

'Never crossed my mind. Could that be why she got Type 2 diabetes later on – isn't there a link?'

'Yes, I'm pretty sure there is.'

Another piece of the jigsaw. If my mother did have gestational diabetes when she was pregnant with me, her blood sugar may well have returned to normal soon after my birth but her likelihood of eventually developing Type 2 diabetes would have been much increased. Taking into account both her eating habits and her ever increasing weight, the odds were well and truly stacked against her.

Children of mothers with gestational diabetes are statistically more likely to become overweight or obese by the time they are teenagers. No one knows exactly why. The glucose levels of blood transferred to the foetus during the pregnancy are altered by the diabetes, but that's not a proven causal link. The link could just as well be the diabetic pregnancy was caused by obesity, with the result that the child is born into a household of overeaters and follows suit.

'It could be at the root of your problems with your weight,' she says.

'It might at least explain why it's been so hard to shift it.'

Information is always helpful but this piece is worrying. Does it mean it's impossible for me to stay out of the obese category? No, surely not. It might make it more difficult – but I refuse to believe it's impossible.

TONIGHT I SPEAK to my brother Crispin in LA, who has just finished training as a therapist. I tell him about this conversation, and how I'm mulling on Bridget and what she means. I ask him for his interpretation of Alcoholics Anonymous's Higher Power. He thinks it can mean whatever you want it to mean, whatever means something useful to you. But he also recognises the idea of an inner voice from other readings, particularly Jung. He compares Bridget's function to the Jungian idea of the 'active imagination'. Reassuringly, he doesn't make me feel mad, or zealous.

Some follow-up research after these conversations produces interesting results. It turns out that a shaman is someone who enters a trance-like state, usually as part of a religious or spiritual ritual, in order to access spirits. The trance is for the purpose of either mental or spiritual healing. But it doesn't quite ring true for me in relation to Bridget.

I have more joy with the idea of the active imagination, developed over a hundred years ago by psychologist Carl Jung as a tool for meditation. He believed there was therapeutic value in creating a bridge between the unconscious and conscious minds by working with dreams and fantasies. The patient would describe scenes which could reveal the workings of the unconscious mind and visualisations of unconscious issues. They would describe images, narratives and characters. Artistic activities such as dance, drama, crafts, music, automatic writing and sculpture could all be used to express the active imagination.

This is closer to Bridget's truth for me. She was a creative idea, a way of telling myself stories that would reveal truths. I have thought of her as either a parable or a meditation. But like all good fictional characters, she has gradually acquired a kind of reality in my mind. I feel I know her, how she thinks, what she might say (if she spoke) and what she's trying to bring to my attention.

That's why it doesn't feel odd when Chris says, 'Why don't you ask Bridget?' It's a kind of shorthand between us for a process that resembles Jung's active imagination.

If I want to know what I really think, that's exactly what I do.

Sobering fact #24: *Obesity in pregnancy has far-reaching implications for the increasing rate of obesity among adolescents and the cycle of obesity in future generations. A relationship between maternal obesity and foetal overgrowth has been noted.*

Journal of Obstetrics and Gynaecology, 2006

CHAPTER 28

Fat is back

Friday, 29 August 2014

IN LONDON THIS week I saw Selina again, super friendly and full of praise for my changing shape. She says I've transformed again since she last saw me.

'You must be a size 10 or 12 now.'

'No, 14, and I've still got a stone to lose.'

'You can't have!'

But I have.

When we part, I visit Bridget to check how she's taken this conversation.

———

Last time Selina showered me with compliments Bridget was livid, stalking around the cave with a right old attitude on her. She thought I was claiming credit that belonged to her.

This time I find her stretched out reading by the fire. I'm surprised, but then notice it's a graphic novel. Well it would be. She always responds to pictures before words.

'Hey you.' We're on more familiar terms these days. 'What did you think of Selina today?'

She gives me an upside-down smile, encouraging but with a sort of 'good-ish' expression.

'Was it was just flattery?'

A shake, not really.

'Does it make any difference to you what people say?' Vehement shake of the head.

'Good. Me neither.'

'Is there any chance I should consider stopping?'

She turns back to her book. Apparently this isn't worthy of reply.

I race down the hillside, buoyant at the difference between this chat and the last, fractious time we talked about Selina.

INCREASING NUMBERS OF people have eating disorders and the media has started to refer to them as 'food addicts'. A recent radio programme on this subject posed questions about the nature of addiction and whether it can be applied to food. A lot less succinct than mine with my brother, by the way.

Overeaters described their obsessive habits: 'I used to go to the fish and chip shop, and buy a battered sausage to eat on the way home as well as my own portion of fish and chips that I would have at home with my family.' 'I eat until I feel literally unable to move' and 'I never ever feel full.' I'm reminded of my own personal favourite: a portion of chips and a Diet Coke. The irony was never lost on me.

The programme featured various forms of treatment including twelve-step programmes, drug therapies which cause nausea if the 'wrong' foods are taken and bariatric surgery which, it implied, should be made more widely available. But the astonishingly missing line of thought in all this was a psychological approach. I know it's hard slog and a slow train, but surely it's bound to be more long-lasting for all that. In my case it's the only route that has ever been really effective. I had to both think and feel my way out of the problem. It's taken time and a lot of guts, if I say so myself, but it wasn't impossible. And for forty years I felt like a lost cause, so if I can do it, anyone can.

For me it's all been about that connection with Bridget, which is another way of saying it's about engaging all parts of the brain. I began by deferring to Bridget and assuming that my verbal self was the lesser partner in decision-making than the unconscious, but I no longer think that. I now understand that the rational self has a duty to strategise and plan ahead.

The hairs on the back of my neck prickle. Suddenly I wonder if this why is we say 'I'm going to start my diet on Monday?' – not because we're being lazy or childish in putting off the evil hour, but because our 'system 2' brains naturally plan ahead. They need time to deliver a message to 'system 1', 'Change of plan! Let's rethink.'

And 'system 1' has a mild case of ADHD because it's always scanning the horizon for danger, and responding to the now. In response, it needs to reconsider its automatic assumptions and adopt a new position.

Maybe I am zealous, as Anna said, but I really can't see how it's possible to tackle addiction without changing the way you think.

ONCE UPON A time there was an accepted wisdom that all changes in the brain take place during childhood, and that by adulthood brains are 'hard-wired'. 'Give me a child until he is seven and I will give you the man,' said Aristotle. No more. Since the mid-twentieth century there's been increasing evidence that the brain is 'plastic', meaning that it continues to change and can self-repair long into maturity.

Norman Doidge's book *The Brain that Changes Itself* relates extraordinary stories of neurologists' interventions to help people 'relearn' lost brain function. One woman had the sensation of constantly falling, even when lying down, due to a loss of function in the vestibular system, which regulates balance. This mechanism works via a set of three semi-circular canals within the inner ear. They are like organic 'spirit levels' consisting of tiny hairs floating in oil which detect horizontal, vertical and directional movement. She had lost 98 per cent of her vestibular function.

To help her relearn to balance, she wore a hat containing an accelerometer which gauged her movements and sent mild electrical signals to a pad on her tongue. These signals mimicked the directions of her body, effectively 'sending balance signals from her tongue to her brain'. At first, she was only able to balance while she wore this equipment, but gradually her brain rediscovered its own vestibular function, and eventually she lost the falling sensation. It took some time but in the end she made an extraordinary recovery.

Doidge's book contains many inspiring stories, like this one, of interventions which were life-changing for sufferers. But they tell us something more: that the brain is subject to change throughout life. It's not over till it's over. You can learn, relearn, change and develop as long as you're still breathing. For those of us with aberrant brains, this is very encouraging news.

More than that, how you use your brain affects the way it develops. Peter and Ellie lived near us in Devon for a few years. He worked at the university researching brain structure while she was a concert pianist. As part of his studies, Peter needed volunteers willing to undergo functional brain scans. He told us what he saw when Ellie agreed to take part and he was able to view his wife's brain in detail.

'As you'd expect, the areas relating to hearing and musicality were large and complex, very well-developed. But her eyes! Her visual centres are just two little dangly bits – it's amazing that she can see anything at all!'

Nature or nurture? Probably both. Presumably Ellie started life with good aural structures in her brain as well as a predisposition to learn, giving her the potential to develop her musicality. But then she spent many hours and years practising and playing, which in turn developed those structures further.

With repetition, our brain structures continue to develop and change. Why should that not apply to recovery from addiction too? My hope is that it does. That continued practice of good dietary habits will win the day and eventually alter my brain so that regulating my weight at a healthy level becomes not an effort but a natural pattern.

TEN YEARS AFTER her diagnosis, my mother was suffering most of the worst side effects of Type 2 diabetes. She was losing her sight. She had neuropathy in both legs, a combination of nerve damage and a circulatory disorder which turned them into unfeeling tree trunks from the knee down. Her hands and feet were numb but painful if touched. The loss of sensation meant that it was hard for her to balance, so she spent most of her time in a chair at home or a wheelchair outside.

In this immobile state she would often dream of running through fields or dancing. She learned ballet from the age of eight to eighteen at Miss Vacani's, a dance school in Kensington. The two little princesses were pupils there too and when she reached the top of the school, from time to time she took them for their bar exercises. 'Of course I taught the Queen to dance,' she would say, airily.

But she was also the woman who in adult life loved to declare, 'The idea of anyone going for a walk for its own sake, with no actual purpose, makes me froth at the mouth with rage.' Not so funny when you think how that turned out.

Physically she deteriorated fast from the age of seventy. Only her voice remained young and vibrant, fresh as ever, telling stories and making jokes, with the result that my two brothers who live abroad had no idea how ill she was getting. I rang them both to let them know.

One said, 'You know what a hypochondriac she is – it's probably nothing.'

'Not this time.' I caught my breath. 'This time, she's not complaining about it. We can all see it.' But her voice had him fooled.

'I don't want to leave you all, but I really do think I've had enough.'

I didn't want her to leave us either. For hours on end, I sat by her chair, voraciously reading, to keep myself from crying, as she dozed beside me.

ONE OF THE major attractions of a low-carb diet is the prediction that it will reduce the risk of diabetes. Within a month or so of starting this regime, however, a *Horizon* programme called 'Sugar v Fat' tests the effects of carb-rich versus fat-rich dieting on the metabolisms of a pair of identical twins.

Astonishingly, by the end of the diet, the twin who ate carbs had significantly healthier insulin resistance than the twin who ate fat. This result is completely counter-intuitive. In theory, if the fat-eating twin carried on with his current eating pattern, he would be at greater risk of diabetes. A sample of two tells us very little and scouring the web I find such a wealth of conflicting information on this subject that I suspect this answer is not yet clear.

I am still convinced from all I've read that fat is not the enemy and that low-carb is the way to go. I carry on, but with my faith shaken in the very aspect of low-carb which most attracted me to this diet.

This is the real diet trap. So many violent opinions, disguised as knowledge, are bandied around that it's very hard to decide on a rational approach. All uttered with certainty, none of it actually certain at all.

WHEN I STARTED out, psychologically it was really hard to stick to a diet, but now it's easy. I've developed that muscle.

On the other hand, physically it was easier. I lost weight then with only minimal effort, but now it's really tough. Still working on that.

Chris strokes my hair. 'I love you through thick and thin,' he says, 'but I prefer thin.'

'Thin' in this context means twelve stone, by the way.

CHAPTER 29

A radical solution

Saturday, 13 September 2014

Bridget and I are going for a slow walk from her tor to the peak of the next one. We are side by side, not touching, rarely looking at each other. We are in step.

'You know what I've been doing of course.' She does.

'You don't disapprove?'

She grins, a quick sideways glance at me telling me that if she disapproved, I wouldn't be doing it.

'Do you think this'll crack it?'

She points at a fox, darting from its cover and streaking off into the distance ahead of us. I think she wants to distract me.

'Pointless question, I suppose. Shall we wait and see?'

We shall.

MOST PEOPLE WITH Type 2 diabetes die of one of three events: a stroke, a heart attack or kidney failure. My mother had a big heart (metaphorically speaking) and I like to think that's why hers lasted, hammering on while the rest of her symptoms raged. The last insult to this great cook and great eater was when she developed diabetic kidney failure. For the last six weeks of her life it robbed her of her appetite, leaving her nauseous and dehydrated, then confused.

Five of her six children were with her, our stepsister too, all waiting and watching.

I find time to talk to her alone.

'Can you carry on without me?'

I nod. My eyes are burning.

Suddenly she's drifting. 'The thing is, I really don't think I can be in the play. Can you put it on without me?'

So life is relegated to a performance. That's so like her.

'Of course. We'll be fine.' I'd like to stroke her hands, but they're numb and painful from the neuropathy, so I don't.

There's one thing I must say to her. And make her understand that I mean it.

'I want you to know how much I love you.'

'Really?' her shoulders sag in what looks like massive relief. Her eyes swim, intensely blue. 'After everything? Really?'

'Yes really.'

Those eyes, blazing with an extraordinary mixture of guilt and shame, love and relief. I'm astonished.

This is the last conversation I ever have alone with her. A day later, just short of her seventy-third birthday, she died.

Dozens of people told us in the days that followed that they personally had had a special bond with her. They rang from all over, came to the house or met us in the street, all saying the same kind of thing – they would always remember what an interest she took in their story, how sympathetic she was, how connected they felt to her. Despite all her flakiness, neediness, absences and drama, her greatest gift was probably her empathy.

But how painful for her to have had that extraordinary quality, and yet to know that she had failed to use it with her own children. To end her life in heartfelt apology.

I had never realised how guilty she felt about me. About all of us. It was heartrending.

*

MY RELATIONSHIP WITH food is completely different from when I started. I don't feel guilty every time I eat, and food is no longer the enemy. I no longer believe that if I go out to dinner and have pudding that I will be five stone heavier in the morning. I've been the same weight for nearly eighteen months, which is about ten pounds over a BMI of 25. I'm a comfortable size 14 and have become easy in my skin here.

Friends and family (but not Chris) tell me that I've done it. They are kind about the transformation. They say I look 'healthy' and 'comfortable', which I'm pretty sure is code for 'thin enough'. I really do appreciate it and I'm not ungrateful, but it's not quite over yet.

At the beginning I recognised that my own body dysmorphia and my troubled past with food meant I was the last person to judge what size or shape I should be, and so I decided to rely on good health guidelines. That's why I used the BMI scale to set myself a target weight. But I haven't quite got there. The chorus of people around me tell me to stop worrying about it but I feel like a member of a relay team who just needs to hand the baton on before I can rest. I aimed at a BMI of 25 so that's where I want to get, even if I end up stabilising a little higher. It's a sense of completion I still need.

'Maybe you just aren't meant to be any less.'

It's amazing the number of people who've said this to me, each offered as if a private insight that I might not have considered myself. I have of course wondered about it, but I go back again and again to the health advice, which suggests I'm still just a little too heavy. That's persuasive enough.

But as I write, I realise that the fixed point of a BMI is not the end of this journey. The place I really need to reach is the end of the lifelong worry about what I eat, a place of ease and relaxation: the End of the Diet. Not yet, but soon, that's still what I'm aiming for.

The next question is what do I need to do differently to lose those last few pounds? A tricky one. In the last three years I've tried the 5:2, the Dukan diet, juicing, 1200 calories a day, low-carb and, of course, WW.

Chris says that every time I've hit a wall on this programme, I've tried something new, or researched a different approach. He thinks persistence is the key and that I've shown I have it. It's great to see how relaxed he is about the whole subject. We both feel we're on the home run.

Two strategies occur to me at once. One is to question my calorie intake. As far as I can tell I've been pretty rigorous in keeping to a regime of around 1200–1300 per day, except for holidays, but since I'm a scratch cook it's sometimes hard to be exact. Could it be that I'm just a little lax, and coupled with occasional days off when I'm eating out, that's enough to stop me losing? If so, one strategy might be to really simplify my diet to basic foods and calorie-counted meals so that I can be exact.

The other way is to choose a meal-replacement programme. As you know, I tried this once before and hated it. It still feels counter to everything I've been trying to do so far. For me, slow dieting is the thing. I also like real food and I'm suspicious of diet products. Finally, I'm scared of this approach because I just don't know if I can do it. I'm not sure that I have the self-control and I'm afraid of trying in case I fail.

Right on cue, there's new research out to show that very low-calorie (known as VLC) diets, including meal replacements, are just as effective long term as a long slow diet. In fact, after three months participants who had used a VLC diet had maintained their weight loss more effectively than the control group.

The system I choose doesn't have glitzy marketing. It was allegedly developed by GPs for 'those who are serious about weight loss'. It takes the form of three milkshakes a day and I soon find they stop me feeling hungry. The worst thing about them is the boredom. But after eight days I've lost four pounds, which is a stunning result.

*

CHRIS NOW TELLS me that he never had any doubt that I would lose weight. He never managed to convey his sense of optimism to me. But to be fair, he did stick with it. He was always trying to get me motivated, although I've advised him not to go for a job as a coach. He's not big on ra-ra.

I worry that I've exposed him through writing so truthfully. There's a note to self on my pad that reads 'Chris – hero or villain?' which is shorthand for this anxiety. His early interventions were sometimes heavy-handed and were certainly painful to hear. I resented the thin bint remark and even more, I thought it was outrageous of him to approach our friends and ask them to support his criticisms about my weight.

But I understand his motivation. He wanted me to live – not for six and half years less than I should, or twenty years less than I should, but for a full healthy lifespan. To him it was obvious that I was curtailing my own life by being seriously overweight. In effect, he staged an intervention.

Would I have got here without him? I have no idea, but I doubt it. What I do know is that I wouldn't have wanted to. And I must add this: no one could have been more generous and supportive in the years that have followed that last painful conversation.

Sobering fact #25: *The average woman in the UK spends thirty-one years of her life dieting.*

Scottish Daily Record, 2007

CHAPTER 30

Set in stones

Friday, 31 October 2014

'Bridget, do you know what you've done for me?'

She's sitting, relaxed, on top of the rock above the cave where I first glimpsed her all those months ago, lurking, peering at me and refusing to come out.

She nods. Of course she does.

'You've allowed me to step away from the problem and look at it from lots of different angles. You've taken the fear out of it. You help me to accept that there are numerous perspectives on these issues but not get overwhelmed by them, or swamped by conflicting pieces of information.'

I suppose I'm thanking her.

'You've shown me how to think about weight. Which is odd, because you're not very cognitive – and not at all verbal.'

She grins. Much less defensive than at the start.

Sometimes I've wished she was a funnier, more attractive alter-ego, one everyone would love. I don't tell her that, of course, and there's a hint of betrayal even in the thought of it. She could have been brighter or more sociable but it's irrelevant. If it was a laugh I wanted, I've got friends for that.

When people ask me what she is, I have to say I don't exactly know. At first I thought she was just a hidden part of my own psyche. I named her so that I could talk to her directly. Even though she doesn't reply, her actions speak louder than words.

But If I close my eyes and concentrate on her, it feels as if she's a source of wisdom and truth which I should cherish, and I do.

An ancient mind indeed.

I WENT TO the doctor this week suffering from some kind of heartburn or indigestion. She said a number of different things could be going on, but first wanted to eliminate heart problems. That was easy because I had an ECG for dental work earlier in the week and it was normal.

'That's alright. But for God's sake if you get short of breath call an ambulance!' Not very reassuring.

She looked at my notes, saw my weight loss and came up with the new theory. She said I might still be producing the same amount of stomach acid as when I was obese, and that with stress (she knows my job is sometimes pressured) adrenaline can surge and push the stomach acid up to the oesophagus, causing a burning sensation. She prescribed digestive medication and told me to stop dieting for a month.

'Stop dieting?' I am anxious at the very thought.

My mind races – I haven't finished yet, I can't risk regaining, it'd be too hard to take it off again, I don't know what 'normal' eating looks like yet.

This is a real challenge. How do I stop dieting?

I have a flashback to a moment just before I began. I was at work and ran downstairs, munching an apple, to chat with one of our company directors. He stood at the bottom of the stairwell looking up at me.

'Eating again?' he said. It's painful having a mirror held up to you with an image of yourself that you don't recognise. I was horrified, stopped in my tracks. Did I really eat all the time? I thought not, but was mortified that it was the impression I gave.

I can't ignore the doctor's advice. I remind myself there's no hurry.

A day or so ago I drove past Cadover Bridge, bathed in afternoon sun. The ice cream van was in situ, lonely as usual in the middle of an empty car park. I drove past, thinking how far I've come.

I will have to stop dieting for a month. What will that look like?

Today the same director ushers me into an edit suite to talk. He wants to read me part of a speech by US President Coolidge.

He says, 'I found this and it made me think of you. "Nothing in this world can take the place of persistence. Talent will not; nothing is more common than unsuccessful men with talent. Genius will not; unrewarded genius is almost a proverb. Education will not; the world is full of educated derelicts. Persistence and determination alone are omnipotent. The slogan Press On! has solved and always will solve the problems of the human race."'

Why he chose this of all moments to share it with me I have no idea, but it couldn't have been more apt.

I tell Chris with some anxiety. What will he make of it? Will he think I'm flaking out? No.

'It's only for a month,' he says. 'And this was all about keeping you healthy anyway – you banana!'

The end, or at least a temporary end, has come quicker than expected. It's been taken out of my hands, but perhaps that's appropriate. Even harder than losing weight is the struggle to give up food anxiety.

CHRIS READS WHAT I've written so far. I ask him if he's happy to be portrayed like this. I worry that it's harsh on him.

'Are you OK with it? Really?'

'Well, it has the benefit of being all true.'

'Good. Thank you.' We're grinning at each other.

Suddenly he looks doubtful. 'There is one thing.' He pauses, a bit self-conscious.

'... I just wish I hadn't used that word.'

'Which one?'

'Bint.'

We both laugh and can't stop.

'I was desperate – I didn't know what to say to motivate you!'

Saturday, 7 February 2015

MY SIXTIETH BIRTHDAY is looming next week and I've made a big push, I've got there. Just. I've arrived at BMI 25.2. By getting back on that horse as soon as my month's rest was over. By chipping away, being resolute and tenacious.

The point is it has taken much longer and the endgame has been much tougher than I ever thought it would be – but it was possible. All those voices in my head saying that it just couldn't be done were rubbish.

My friend Tim comes into the room as we're laying out food for the party. I have my back to him. He comes up behind me and pats me on the shoulder.

'I wondered who that was, standing at the table. I didn't recognise you.'

'But you saw me yesterday!'

'Yes, but suddenly you looked like a stranger.' He grins. I've done well.

It takes one very small step in front of another. It takes being pleased with minimal amounts of progress. I'm not talking about weight loss here, but being at peace with myself about food. Getting rid of the cavilling lodger in my head who was always ready to keep up a negative running commentary on my daily intake.

Towards the end of the evening, I cut the cake. I think of all those AA cakes, made to celebrate sobriety birthdays. This can be my sobriety cake, but privately.

I still feel embarrassed that it matters. I still think that there are far more important things to worry about. But this is one worry that I no longer have to fight with.

It's taken me all these years, until I was nearly sixty, to recognise the addictive nature of my eating habits and the strong streak of denial running through my thinking. I've learned to accept that addictive behaviour is part of who I am. So, if I eat a lot one day, I cut back the next. I'm sometimes still surprised that after such lapses I don't wake up six stone heavier, but I don't.

It makes me tired to think how much of my life I've wasted thinking anxiously about food. And what good did all that anxiety do me? Did it mean I learned to live with it, and conquer my problematic eating habits? Of course it didn't.

Until now ...! That's what a real diet book would say ... Until now ... grand revelation!! I've solved it, readers! Come with me. I've seen the light and I'm going to shine it on you too.

Except you know, really you do, that it's not like that. This is not a one size fits all solution. It's slow, sometimes painful, stolid, faltering and repetitive, frequently feels as though it's losing its way, remains steady-ish, battles on and stumbles through.

But the great good news is this – gets there in the end. Promise. Gets there in the end.

CHAPTER 31

Cadover Bridget

2017

I come less often to see Bridget these days. She's there, but there's nothing urgent to say. We're not in fractious dispute the way we once were.

'Bridget, in the end, was it all about brain chemistry?'

She almost smiles. As if to say 'it was – and it wasn't'.

'I see, so even if it was about mood and emotion, that translates into brain chemistry too …'

But she's gone, striding up to the top of the tor to gaze out across the landscape. Reminding me of my sister Belinda.

'Are you still going on about that?' she seems to be saying.

⌁

THE TEST OF success is not the last weigh-in at the end of a diet but in the longevity of the weight loss.

Given what we know about the boomerang effect, i.e. that weight loves to come bouncing back, in greater quantity than was there in the first place, here I am checking in, three years on, still within spitting distance of where I was then.

It's been twelve years since that distant moment of revelation at Cadover Bridge and six years since I dreamed up Bridget. Cadover Bridget, she should be called.

These days I practise what I call 'astral dieting'. It comes from a game Orlando and I used to play when he was very small and extremely ticklish. I would raise my hand just above his body and make as if to tickle, without touching. He would collapse in giggles. This was astral tickling. The further away from him I could hold my hands and still make him laugh, the more satisfying it was. The tickling was all in the mind.

Astral dieting has no points, no counting, no specific foods, no regime – because it too is all in the mind. It's an inner knowledge of what I need to eat to stay on track. But to be fair, I learned this through counting. When a child learns the piano, she uses a metronome to help her hold the beat. By grade 8 she can read music, including its rhythm. That's what I've done. It's not always perfect but for the three years since I made that last push it's kept me within a couple of points of BMI 25. We are told that 97 per cent of dieters regain all their lost weight and more within three years. I've bucked the stats.

There are no claims of permanent weight loss here. I consider myself, like a recovered alcoholic, only a bite away from slipping back into bad old ways. But six years on from starting, this project speaks for itself. The longer I stay here, the more likely it is that I will take up residence. I plan to move my 'set point', that 12 to 15 pound spectrum that the body naturally shifts up and down, once and for all. I'm hoping for squatters' rights in the normal weight range.

And I can clearly say that I've recovered from the Cadover Bridge Syndrome: I don't eat unconsciously any more. That was a huge issue which made me doubt my own sanity. Through a combination of mindful eating and self-education, I've learned to stay in the moment, which is a great relief.

This is the best bit: when I began, I had a one in three risk of developing Type 2 diabetes. Given my age and the fact that my mother had Type 2 diabetes, my background risk (the best odds I can achieve) is one in ten. And that's where I am now: one in ten (drifting, occasionally, to one in eight, but no worse). Higher than I would like it, but pretty much as low as it can be. I set out to push the risk as far away from me as I could, and I've done it.

So how? After all that effort, what was it that worked and made it possible for me to lose weight when I hadn't been able to for all those years before?

The National Weight Control Study in Rhode Island was set up in 1994 to chart successful dieters. Recognising the prevailing impression that diets fail, and losers regain, the intention was to recruit people who had lost at least thirty pounds and kept it off for a year or more and to study their success.

Perhaps surprisingly, their findings show a huge range of ways that people on the register have lost weight. Nearly half did it on their own, while the rest were members of a weight loss programme. Almost all modified their food intake and a very high proportion increased their physical activity, the most popular activity reported being walking.

Over more than twenty years, here are some common elements that people on the National Weight Control Registry have used to regulate their weight:

- 78 per cent eat breakfast every day.
- 75 per cent weigh themselves at least once a week.
- 62 per cent watch less than ten hours of TV per week.
- 90 per cent exercise, on average, about 1 hour per day.

In other words, there isn't one simple technique or regime. There are multiple approaches that help. In the end, hard work and perseverance win the day.

By instinct I used a patchwork of methods too, just like the people on the register, including different diets and exercise. I educated myself, as much as I could, about the causes and potential treatments for obesity.

At the outset, I decided to regard it as a project and try to take the emotion out of it. As it turned out, it is probably more accurate to say that I separated out the emotion from all the other issues in play. For a long time I treated it like a puzzle or a cognitive problem. That was very effective and it got me most of the way, but in the end I had to deal with the emotional issues around food too. That's what makes weight loss so hard. There's so much going on – physical, mental, emotional and societal factors all bringing pressure to bear. It's a right old muddle and it needs a lot thinking through.

Finally, of course, there was talking to Bridget. She saw me through it all. Considering that she's fictional, she's been an enormous help. She challenged me, encouraged me, comforted and educated me. And always made me laugh. It was a relief to have her sardonic input to this knotty old problem.

It's through talking to Bridget that I learned to stop eating unconsciously. She helped me to stay in the moment, and that's where I need to be.

AN ADMISSION: IT took me years to stop paying money to WW even when I wasn't using the programme, the food or weight-logging systems. A kind of crazy superstition stopped me from bowing out. Chris would see the transaction on the credit card and raise an eyebrow.

'You really don't need this. Why?'

'Because. It's not much. Think of it as an obesity tax.'

'But you're not obese. Mad woman.'

And this is a real issue in dieting. We, the dieting population (and that's most of us), are sitting duck consumers for diet products, special foods, media of all sorts and celebrity narratives which appear to offer solutions to obesity but in fact work on ever-replicating need, rather than a satisfactory end point.

Karl Marx had a phrase for it: commodity fetishism. We are drawn to diet products because we see only what they purport to offer. That is, the hope of transformation; in effect, a belief system. But far from actually offering that transformation, the economic model works by maintaining our addiction to dieting as a replacement for our addiction to food.

I've given up both. I'm a recovered obesenic and a recovering dietaholic.

I USED TO think that my parents were idealists with feet of clay. Their good intentions to change the world were excellent, but looked at in close-up they failed to deliver on a fairly spectacular scale. There's a line from the musical *Hair* which always make me think of them:

'Do you only care about the bleeding crowd? How about a needing friend?'

They believed that they had answers to child-rearing that no one else had, especially in the restrictive post-war period. At that time, state schools were like borstals and public schools (where they had gone) were recruitment centres for the forces, politics or the debutante circuit. They talked persuasively about their vision of a perfect therapeutic community at their school. They were particularly hot on the rights of children. Theoretically.

'People like us ought to have children,' my mother would declare. I was three when I first questioned that certainty. I didn't know the word arrogant, but if I had, that's what I would have called it.

In fact, to call it 'feet of clay' is mealy-mouthed. There was more straightforward neglect in it than that. We were grubby, dishevelled children with dirt under our fingernails, not made to brush our teeth for fear of restricting our freedom, barefoot as a matter of pride. We were also free, very free, in a way that would be exceptional now but was positively outlandish then. We were also abandoned, both physically and emotionally, by each of them in turn.

What were they thinking of, getting us lost in fog, at night, in the middle of France, with no money, no food, no shelter? Not just us, but a lorry load of children in care that they were responsible for? Sheer madness.

Particularly confusing is that, despite everything, I loved and admired them both so much. It's taken a lot of therapy to unpick that.

*

THESE DAYS MY mantra is this: food is just food. It's not an emotional issue. It's not comfort or joy, companionship or calm. Food is just food.

A FEW DAYS ago, I was heading towards Cadover Bridge on my way home from work. It was the hottest day for forty years and the ice cream van was certain to be there.

On this sweltering afternoon, I consciously made the decision to stop and buy a (calorifically cheap) ice lolly to cool myself down. My car swept over the hill and I gazed down at the heaving car park, the ice cream van sitting in the middle of row upon row of cars, all glinting in the sunshine. People were picnicking along the river bank, having come to take a dip in the welcoming icy waters of the fast-flowing River Plym. I looked for a spot where I could pull in.

My car approached the entrance gap but I didn't signal or slow down. In fact I didn't turn off at all, but drove on towards home with no cooling Mivvi in my hand.

'Hello, Bridget,' I said, grinning to myself. 'Still at it, I see.'

Just when you think you've made a clear, mindful decision, which is perfectly alright and does not disrupt your regime in any damaging way, your inner self takes you down another path, showing once again who's the boss of who. Bridget obviously took the view that whenever you can resist eating something unnecessary and not nutritious, you should. But it's Bridget who made that decision, not me.

I laugh, but I'm grateful. Bridget and I are no longer at war. This is not a difference of opinion which makes me question my sanity, as it once did, but instead makes me feel as though I've found it.

Afterword

'Bridget, are there any words of wisdom you want to share?'

A shrug, a grunt. As if.

'Well, do you know why I picked you? Why not Marina, the mermaid? I liked the sound of her.'

She laughs, actually laughs.

'I see. So I didn't pick you at all? It was you, you did the picking?'

Of course it was.

Who else?

The slow diet manifesto

This is my manifesto for slow dieting:

1. Do the mental work

The biggest help you can give yourself is to be your own detective. Work through your history and your present to see what drives you. Be truthful about it but also be forgiving. Learn to be flexible and accept solutions which are far from perfect. Train yourself to succeed.

2. Do it slowly

At least at the beginning. It's easier for you to carry out. It's likely to be more permanent. It's less of a shock to your system. It gives your skin a chance to recover and shrink in line with your weight loss, leaving no sagging folds of loose flesh. If you want to speed up in the later stages, so be it.

3. Keep it balanced

We are omnivores and should eat like omnivores, a little of everything, nothing forbidden. Rules that are too strict are hard to keep.

4. Keep it varied

If a diet stops working, change it. We are not cult members. Just because we joined one diet programme, it is not our failure if it stops working. Feel free to move on.

5. Set a realistic timeframe for changing your diet, but no timetable for your weight loss

It will take as long as it takes. A year is a good place to start. Once that time is over, the second year is easy to commit to. If you have a lot to lose, you will be very lucky to shed as much as a pound a week long term, whatever the magazines tell you.

6. Practise patience

This is a long slow process. Calm your thinking and ease yourself into it. This will help when weight is slow to shift, or when inevitable plateaus hit.

7. Practise restraint

Teach yourself to wait a while between desire and consumption. Stretch the waiting time. It's a habit you can learn. You are not helpless over your own behaviour.

8. Sleep

Recognise that lack of sleep is associated with obesity and commit to resting for eight hours a night, and getting as much sleep as possible in that time.

9. Treat diet products cautiously

Eat normal food and use portion control to restrict calories. A few judiciously chosen diet products may be helpful. But be aware that there is often very little calorie difference between a diet product and the non-diet version. 'Low fat' versions often have added carbs or sugars to make them more palatable.

10. Chart your progress

Measure success in the long term, not daily or weekly. Half a pound off a week sounds like a minimal result, but half a stone in three months sounds great. They're the same thing. Commit for the long term.

11. Give yourself recovery time

At the end of your diet you will need to allow at least half as much time again to regularise your calorie intake and adjust to your new weight. Factor it in right from the start so that you don't trip up at the end.

12. Learn to say yes

It's as important to say yes as to say no to our own desires. Don't make this process a torment. Sometimes consciously decide to relax the diet regime in a positive way – not a lapse, but a decision. Eat mindfully. Enjoy this moment to the full, and then practise restraint afterwards.

Reading list

Thinking, Fast and Slow by Daniel Kahneman
Fat is a Feminist Issue by Susie Orbach
The Brain that Changes Itself by Norman Doidge
The Dukan Diet by Dr Pierre Dukan
The Fast Diet by Dr Michael Mosley
Escape the Diet Trap by Dr John Briffa
Why We Get Fat by Gary Taubes
The F-Plan Diet by Audrey Eyton
Dr Atkins' New Diet Revolution by Robert C. Atkins

And other media

'Neuroscience', *In Our Time*, BBC Radio 4, 13 Nov 2008: http://www.bbc.co.uk/programmes/b00fbd26

'Why Dieting Doesn't Usually Work', Sandra Aamodt, TED Talk, 8 Jan 2014: https://www.ted.com/talks/sandra_aamodt_why_dieting_doesn_t...

Sobering facts and other studies

Chapter 1

Sobering fact #1: Over 63 per cent of Brits and 70 per cent of Americans are overweight.

National Statistics, 'Health Survey for England, 2015', NHS Digital, 14 December 2016

https://digital.nhs.uk/catalogue/PUB22610

Cheryl D. Fryar, et al., 'Prevalence of overweight, obesity, and extreme obesity among adults aged 20 and over: United States, 1960–1962 through 2013–2014', National Center for Health Statistics, July 2016

https://www.cdc.gov/nchs/data/hestat/obesity_adult_13_14/obesity_adult_13_14.htm

Chapter 2

'Recent studies have described soup as an aid to dieting because it gives a sense of fullness without a big calorie load.'

Jack Challoner, 'How soup can help you lose weight', BBC News Magazine, 26 May 2009

http://news.bbc.co.uk/1/hi/magazine/8068733.stm

Sobering fact #2: 26 per cent of British people and 36 per cent of Americans are obese, which means they have a BMI over 30.

National Statistics, 'Statistics on obesity, physical activity and diet – England, 2016', NHS Digital, 28 April 2016

https://digital.nhs.uk/catalogue/PUB20562

Cynthia L. Ogden, et al., 'Prevalence of obesity among adults and youth: United States 2011–2014', National Center for Health Statistics, November 2015

https://www.cdc.gov/nchs/data/databriefs/db219.pdf

Chapter 3

Sobering fact #3. Currently, 90 per cent of adults with Type 2 diabetes are overweight or obese. People with severe obesity are at greater risk of Type 2 diabetes than obese people with a lower BMI.

Gatineau Mary, et al, 'Adult obesity and Type 2 Diabetes', Public Health England, July 2014

https://www.gov.uk/government/uploads/system/uploads/attachment_data/file/338934/Adult_obesity_and_type_2_diabetes_.pdf

Chapter 4

'Here's an exercise which combines distress tolerance and mindfulness'

Elisha Carcieri, 'DBT skills for eating disorders', Eating Disorder Therapy LA, 5 April 2016

https://www.eatingdisordertherapyla.com/dbt-skills-for-eating-disorders/

Sobering fact #4: 29 million people in the UK tried to lose weight in 2013.

Mintel, 'Dieting in 2014? You're not alone', 3 January 2014

http://www.mintel.com/press-centre/social-and-lifestyle/dieting-in-2014-you-are-not-alone

Chapter 5

Sobering fact #5: Most diets claim weight loss of 1–2 pounds per week is achievable, but research shows this is an unrealistic expectation.

National Institutes of Health, 'NIH research model predicts weight with varying diet, exercise changes', 25 August 2011 https://www.nih.gov/news-events/news-releases/nih-research-model-predicts-weight-varying-diet-exercise-changes

Chapter 6

Sobering fact #6: The global weight loss industry was worth $176 billion in 2017. And yet obesity rates continue to rise.

Research and Markets, 'Weight loss and weight management market by equipment, surgical equipment, diet, and weight loss services', October 2017

https://www.researchandmarkets.com/reports/4416739/weight-loss-and-weight-management-market-by

Chapter 7

Sobering fact #7: More men are overweight or obese than women. In 2015, 68 per cent of men in the UK were overweight or obese compared with 58 per cent of women.

House of Commons Library, 'Obesity statistics', 20 January 2017

http://researchbriefings.parliament.uk/ResearchBriefing/Summary/SN03336

Chapter 8

Sobering fact #8: 'Weight watching' is by no means female territory anymore – 65 per cent of women and 44 per cent of men in Britain tried to lose weight in 2013.

Mintel, 'Dieting in 2014? You're not alone', 3 January 2014

http://www.mintel.com/press-centre/social-and-lifestyle/dieting-in-2014-you-are-not-alone

Chapter 9

'"The evidence suggests that you would be more likely to select the tempting chocolate cake when your mind is loaded with digits. System 1 has more influence on behaviour when system 2 is busy, and it has a sweet tooth."'

Daniel Kahneman, *Thinking, Fast and Slow*, Allen Lane, 2011

Sobering fact #9: Parent weight change is related to child weight change. Family-based behavioural treatments are among the most successful for paediatric obesity while parental obesity may increase the risk of a child becoming obese.

Brian H. Wrotniak, et al., 'Parent weight change as a predictor of child weight change in family-based behavioral obesity treatment', *JAMA Paediatrics*, April 2004

https://jamanetwork.com/journals/jamapediatrics/fullarticle/485676

Chapter 10

'£5000–£15,000 for a stomach staple, gastric bypass or gastric band'

In the UK, bariatric surgeries increased by 530 per cent over five years, rising to over six thousand surgeries in 2012–2013.

NHS Choices, 'Gastric bypass surgery "up 530% in 6 years"', 24 August 2012

https://www.nhs.uk/news/obesity/gastric-bypass-surgery-up-530-in-6-years/

Sobering fact #10: In 2000, about 37,000 bariatric surgeries were performed in the United States. By 2013, the number had risen to 220,000.

Harriet Brown, *Body of Truth: How Science, History and Culture Drive our Obsession with Weight*, De Capo, 2015

Chapter 11

'Both groups lost weight, but the technology-free set lost nearly twice as much (13lb versus 7.7lb) as those who scrutinised every step electronically.'

Prof Eric A. Finkelstein, et al., 'Effectiveness of activity trackers with and without incentives to increase physical activity', *The Lancet, Diabetes & Endocrinology*, 4 October 2016

http://www.thelancet.com/journals/landia/article/PIIS2213-8587(16)30284-4/abstract

Sobering fact #11: Overweight and obese children are significantly more likely to be obese in adulthood.

World Health Organization, 'Facts and figures on childhood obesity', 13 October 2017

http://www.who.int/end-childhood-obesity/facts/en/

Chapter 12

'we are all more suggestible than previously thought.'

Andrew K. Przybylski and Netta Weinstein, 'Can you connect with me now? How the presence of mobile communication technology influences face-to-face conversation quality', *Journal of Social and Personal Relationships*, 19 July 2012

http://journals.sagepub.com/doi/abs/10.1177/0265407512453827

Sobering fact #12: Research in both the UK and the US is emerging to show that exercise has a negligible impact on weight loss.

Emma John, 'Why exercise won't make you thin', *Observer*, 19 September 2010

https://www.theguardian.com/lifeandstyle/2010/sep/19/exercise-dieting-public-health

Mintel, 'Dieting in 2014? You're not alone', 3 January 2014

http://www.mintel.com/press-centre/social-and-lifestyle/dieting-in-2014-you-are-not-alone

Chapter 13

'One study tested the effect of injecting leptin into twenty-seven women whose weight had plateaued after bariatric surgery.'

X. Terra, et al., 'Long-term changes in leptin, chemerin and ghrelin levels following bariatric surgery procedures', *Obesity Surgery*, 23 November 2013

https://www.ncbi.nlm.nih.gov/pubmed/23832521

Sobering fact #13: Holidays seem to increase body weight in adults. Participants seeking to lose weight appeared to increase weight over the holiday period.

Rolando G. Díaz-Zavala, et al., 'Effect of the holiday season on weight gain', *Journal of Obesity*, 4 July 2017

https://www.hindawi.com/journals/jobe/2017/2085136/

Chapter 14

Sobering fact #14: It is difficult to maintain weight loss. Contestants on *The Biggest Loser* lost an average of 127lb each but over time thirteen of fourteen gained 66 per cent of the weight lost.

Erin Fothergill, et al., 'Persistent metabolic adaptation 6 years after "The Biggest Loser" competition', *Obesity*, 2 May 2016

http://onlinelibrary.wiley.com/doi/10.1002/oby.21538/full

Alexandra Sifferlin, 'The weight loss trap: why your diet isn't working', *Time*, 25 May 2017

http://time.com/magazine/us/4793878/june-5th-2017-vol-189-no-21-u-s/

Chapter 15

Sobering fact #15: In the UK, we spend over £11 billion a year on care of Type 2 diabetes and its complications.

Panos Kanavos, et al., 'Diabetes expenditure, burden of disease and management in 5 EU countries', LSE Health, London School of Economics, January 2012

http://www.lse.ac.uk/LSEHealthAndSocialCare/research/LSEHealth/MTRG/LSE_Diabetes_EXECSUM_24JAN2012.pdf

Chapter 16

Sobering fact #16. An analysis of 57,000 women in 2013 found that those who experienced physical or sexual abuse as children were twice as likely to be addicted to food than those who did not.

Susan M. Mason, et al., 'Abuse victimization in childhood or adolescence and risk of food addiction in adult women', *Obesity*, 29 July 2013

http://onlinelibrary.wiley.com/doi/10.1002/oby.20500/
abstract?isLogout=true

Chapter 17

'I see an article in the *Daily Mail* declaring that the best way to help your child lose weight is to lose it yourself'

Brian H. Wrotniak, et al., 'Parent weight change as a predictor of child weight change in family-based behavioral obesity treatment', *JAMA Paediatrics*, April 2004

https://jamanetwork.com/journals/jamapediatrics/fullarticle/485676

'I had never heard of "sleep obesity" until now, but Dr Eve Van Cauter has a doctorate in it.'

Eve Van Cauter, et al., 'The impact of sleep deprivation on hormones and metabolism', *Medscape Neurology*, 2005

https://www.medscape.org/viewarticle/502825

Sebastian M. Schmid, et al., 'A single night of sleep deprivation increases ghrelin levels and feelings of hunger in normal-weight healthy men', *Journal of Sleep Research*, 29 June 2008

http://onlinelibrary.wiley.com/doi/10.1111/j.1365-2869.2008.00662.x/full

Kristen L. Knutson, et al., 'The metabolic consequences of sleep deprivation', *Sleep Medical Reviews*, June 2007

http://www.smrv-journal.com/article/S1087-0792(07)00020-2/fulltext

Sobering fact #17: When stressed, our body goes into survival mode: Cortisol, the 'stress hormone', is secreted, which can cause an increase in appetite.

Harvard Health Publishing, 'Understanding the stress response', March 2011

https://www.health.harvard.edu/staying-healthy/understanding-the-stress-response

Chapter 18

Sobering fact #18: Having previously been on a diet has been determined as a predictor of weight gain.

Michael R. Lowe, et al., 'Dieting and restrained eating as prospective predictors of weight gain', *Frontiers in Psychology*, 2 September 2013

https://www.ncbi.nlm.nih.gov/pmc/articles/PMC3759019/

Chapter 19

Sobering fact #19: An estimated 7.1 per cent of deaths (35,820) are attributable to elevated BMI in England and Wales in 2014. Each individual lost twelve years on average.

Mark Tovey, 'Obesity and the public purse', Institute of Economic Affairs discussion paper No. 80, January 2017

https://iea.org.uk/wp-content/uploads/2017/01/Obesity-and-the-Public-Purse-PDF.pdf

Chapter 20

Sobering fact #20: 80 per cent French women are thought to be on a diet at any given time.

Gabrielle Deydier, *On ne naît pas grosse*, Goutte d'or, 2017

Stefanie Marsh, 'Gabrielle Deydier – what it's like to be fat in France', *Observer*, 10 September 2017

https://www.theguardian.com/society/2017/sep/10/gabrielle-deydier-fat-in-france-abuse-grossophobia-book-women

Chapter 21

'Brain activity consumes a disproportionate amount of energy at 20 per cent of our BMR'

Ferris Jabr, 'Does thinking really hard burn more calories?', *Scientific American*, 18 July 2012

https://www.scientificamerican.com/article/thinking-hard-calories/

Sobering fact #21: 'Obesity is the new smoking, and it represents a slow-motion car crash in terms of avoidable illness and rising health care cost.'

Simon Stevens, CEO NHS England at the Public Health England annual conference, quoted in Nick Triggle, 'Obesity is the new smoking, says NHS boss in England', BBC News, 2014

http://www.bbc.co.uk/news/health-29253071

Chapter 23

'I've seen plenty of studies claiming the ketogenic diets are safe and promote long-term weight loss more effectively than other low-carb diets. However, a study reported in the *American Journal of Clinical Nutrition* in 2006 . . .'

Marcelo Campos, 'Ketogenic diet: Is the ultimate low-carb diet good for you?' Harvard Health Publishing, Harvard Medical School, 27 July 2017

https://www.health.harvard.edu/blog/ketogenic-diet-is-the-ultimate-low-carb-diet-good-for-you-2017072712089

C.S. Johnston, et al., 'Ketogenic low-carbohydrate diets have no metabolic advantage over nonketogenic low-carbohydrate diets', *American Journal of Clinical Nutrition*, May 2006

https://www.ncbi.nlm.nih.gov/pubmed/16685046

'I'm encouraged by an item on the radio claiming that Type 2 diabetes can be reversed by a very low-calorie diet.'

Michael E.J. Lean, et al., 'Primary care-led weight management for remission of Type 2 diabetes', *The Lancet*, 5 December 2017

http://www.thelancet.com/journals/lancet/article/PIIS0140-6736(17)33102-1/fulltext

Chapter 25

'"Compulsive eaters crave their food as badly as a junkie craves heroin . . ."'

Susie Orbach, *Fat is a Feminist Issue*, Paddington Press, 1978 (now published by Arrow)

'There's news this morning that as part of a response to the obesity crisis, bariatric surgery is going to be made more easily available.'

Owen Haskins, 'UK needs 50,000 bariatric procedures a year', Bariatric News, 12 May 2016

http://www.bariatricnews.net/?q=news/112378/uk-needs-50000-bariatric-procedures-year

Sobering fact #22: A group of 105 women who received cognitive therapy lost more weight and kept it off over the next 18 months, while those assigned to a waiting list for therapy gained weight over the same period.

L. Stahre and T. Hallstrom, 'A short-term cognitive group treatment program gives substantial weight reduction up to 18 months from the end of treatment', *Journal of Eating and Weight Disorders*, March 2005

https://www.ncbi.nlm.nih.gov/pubmed/15943172

Chapter 26

'Now scientists have discovered what they are calling "beige" fat.'

Endocrine Society, 'Cold exposure prompts body to convert white fat to calorie-burning beige fat', 2014

https://www.endocrine.org/news-room/press-release-archives/2014/cold-exposure-prompts-body-to-convert-white-fat-to-calorie-burning-beige-fat

'Another simple technique to aid weight loss is to turn our household heating down.'

Stephen Cousins, 'Some like it hot: Dynamic temperatures boost health', *RIBJ*, 12 May 2017

https://www.ribaj.com/products/research-health-maastricht-university-medical-centre-environment-temperature

Sobering fact #23: In the UK, about £6 billion a year is spent on the direct medical costs of conditions related to being overweight or obese. A further £10 billion is spent on diabetes.

McKinsey & Company, 'Overcoming obesity – An initial economic analysis', November 2014 http://affinityhealthhub.co.uk/storage/app/attachments/mgi-overcoming-obesity-full-report-2014-1488562931.pdf

Chapter 27

'Sugar is the new bad guy in town'

William T. Basco, Jr, 'Sucrose analgesia for infants: State of the science', *Medscape*, 17 December 2010, commentary on D. Harrison, et al., 'Analgesic effects of sweet-tasting solutions for infants', *Pediatrics*, 2010

https://www.medscape.com/viewarticle/733969?src=trendmd_pilot

B. Stevens, et al., 'Sucrose for analgesia (pain relief) in newborn infants undergoing painful procedures', *Cochrane*, 15 July 2016

http://www.cochrane.org/CD001069/NEONATAL_sucrose-analgesia-pain-relief-newborn-infants-undergoing-painful-procedures

'"I've always wondered if mum's pregnancy with you was diabetic, because the rest of us were much lighter at birth – around seven to eight pounds, which is more normal."'

Matthew W. Gillman, et al., 'Maternal gestational diabetes, birth weight, and adolescent obesity', *Pediatrics*, March 2003

http://pediatrics.aappublications.org/content/111/3/e221.short

Salynn Boyles, 'Gestational diabetes ups child obesity', *WebMD*, 28 August 2007

https://www.webmd.com/baby/news/20070828/gestational-diabetes-ups-child-obesity#1

Sobering fact #24: Obesity in pregnancy has far-reaching implications for the increasing rate of obesity among adolescents and the cycle of obesity in future generations. A relationship between maternal obesity and foetal overgrowth has been noted.

P.M. Catalano and H.M. Ehrenberg, 'The short- and long-term implications of maternal obesity on the mother and her offspring', *Journal of Obstetrics and Gynaecology*, October 2006

https://www.ncbi.nlm.nih.gov/pubmed/16827826

Chapter 29

'there's new research out to show that very low-calorie (known as VLC) diets, including meal replacements, are just as effective long term as a long slow diet.'

Katrina Purcell, et al., 'The effect of rate of weight loss on long-term weight management', *The Lancet: Diabetes & Endocrinology*, 15 October 2014

http://www.thelancet.com/journals/landia/article/PIIS2213-8587(14)70200-1/abstract

Sobering fact #25: The average woman in the UK spends thirty-one years of her life dieting.

Natalie Walker, 'The 31 year diet', *Scottish Daily Record*, 24 January 2007

https://www.dailyrecord.co.uk/news/uk-world-news/the-31-year-diet-947696

Chapter 31

'The National Weight Control Study in Rhode Island was set up in 1994 to chart successful dieters.'

National Weight Control Registry, 'NWCR facts', accessed January 2018

http://www.nwcr.ws/Research/default.htm

Acknowledgements

I'VE HAD A great deal of help writing this book and I am grateful to many people for their encouragement, support and feedback, not to mention endless coffees.

First, I'd like to thank Julie Myerson, Debbie Taylor, Jenny Brown and Jane Martinson, the judging panel who chose an early draft of the book for the *Mslexia* Memoir Award 2014. It was a huge surprise and gave me a massive boost of confidence at that delicate stage of writing.

Thanks to my agent, Julian Alexander, for keeping faith with the idea through its long gestation, and to Hannah MacDonald and Charlotte Cole from September Publishing who helped to usher it into being. Their editorial insight has been invaluable.

My friends and family were my first readers and offered lots of advice and enthusiasm. They also insisted on a few deletions, which is probably just as well. Thanks to Joe Ahearne, Nicole Cauverien, Roopa Gulati, Barbara Freeman, Jill Hitchins, Suki Hughes, Janet Burgess, Julia Keen, Crispin Kitto, Miranda Scholefield and all my lovely colleagues at Denhams.

My medical friends are due particular thanks for helping to steer me towards some semblance of factual accuracy when I strayed into areas beyond my knowledge. Thanks to Simon Freeman, Sarah Adams and Charlie Lloyd. Special thanks to Alice Adams for help with research.

I'm grateful to my friends Vicky Burnard, consultant clinical psychologist and specialist in eating disorders, Anthony Venditti, existential therapist and clinical supervisor, and

Hilary Prentice, psychotherapist and ecopsychotherapist, all of whom have generously given their time and made suggestions which have helped shape the final draft. Thanks to Professor David Papineau for kindly replying to my emails and then even more kindly allowing me to reproduce them here.

And of course, thanks to Chris and Orlando: for reading it (many times), listening to me going on about it, propping me when spirits flagged and giving me the courage to keep at it. What a pair.

About the author

GRACE KITTO IS a TV producer who lives in Devon with her husband and son. This is her first book. An early draft won the *Mslexia* Memoir Award 2014.

"Saving Sandra"

1. Began in earnest on Mon 7 Oct 2019.